Expansion

THE JOURNEY CONTINUES

The sequel to

Enclosure:

A SPIRITUAL AUTOBIOGRAPHY

BARBARA BECKER

Editing by The Pro Book Editor
Interior and Cover Design by IAPS.rocks

eBook ISBN: 978-0-9787700-3-7
paperback ISBN: 978-0-9787700-2-0

     1. Main category—General Biography & Autobiography
     2. Other category—New Age & Spirituality

First Edition

BOOKS BY BARBARA BECKER

Enclosure: A Spiritual Autobiography

Expansion: The Journey Continues

Time Travels: Exploration of Lives Remembered

I dedicate this book to my Higher Self,
the collective of beings from the Great
Central Sun known as the WhiteOne.

TABLE OF CONTENTS

INTRODUCTION

by James Martin Peebles, MD (1822-1922)
channeled through Barbara Becker

G OD BLESS YOU INDEED! DR. Peebles here! It's a pleasure and a joy when man and Spirit come together in the search for greater truth and awareness. Yah, dear Barbara, you have touched the face of God in your lifetime of experiences. How wonderful that you are sharing you with the world—all of the ups and downs, nooks and crannies of Barbara—and nothing less! In this reveal and revelation of your journey to the heart, you give inspiration for those searching for their truth and their love to discover it was all inside of them in the first place.

You asked us years ago if you wrote a book and shared your understandings, and those understandings changed in the future, would you need to write another book? Well, dear Barbara, this was that book—a demonstration of expanding your mind and your heart. Just as God continues to experience and learn from further experiences, so do each and every one of you. So, yes, we spoke of two books, and this completes that conversation because you have changed from the enclosure of who you were to the expansion of who you are now. You, my dear, have set yourself free. It was a grand and glorious realization to behold and witness. God bless you indeed, dear Barbara!

The readers of your book will find further inspiration for their own journeys. They learn so much from your experiences and how you faced your challenges. Changing one's perspective was the greatest healer of all, as you know and have learned. Yes, your wisdom that lies deep within you does come from the lifetime you had as a Tibetan monk. It was no error that others are drawn to you because you have knowledge and the intellect to present esoteric concepts in terms others would understand. God bless you indeed!

PROLOGUE

F ROM 1963 TO 1969, MY family's summer vacations consisted of camping from Florida to Upstate New York, visiting relatives in the Adirondack area where I was born in 1955. In the early years, we camped in a four-wall tent that was large enough for adults to stand up. We graduated to a pop-up tent trailer that slept four people, and my brothers slept in a separate two-person tent. This was an upgrade from sleeping bags on the ground with a cot or air mattresses inflated with a foot pump.

When I was twelve years old, camping in the Great Smokey Mountains of Tennessee, I walked down the hill at dusk from our campsite to the public restroom to brush my teeth before bed. As I walked out of the ladies' room, I saw a dark object about six inches in front of me, moving from left to right. As my eyes came into focus, I realized I was staring at the back end of a black bear. Our paths just happened to cross as the bear was on his way to the parking lot garbage cans. It was 1967, and the trash cans were above ground and easily rummaged by hungry bears looking for leftover scraps of food. This was not a baby bear nor a full-sized adult. With Goldilocks's perception, the bear was the right size to scare the wits out of me. The back of the bear's behind was at the level of my waist.

I screamed as I jumped out of my flip-flops and ran up the path. The bear was startled by my scream, quickening his pace toward the parking lot. A woman in her thirties standing at the back end of her station wagon looked in my direction. She saw the bear running toward her, jumped on the top of her car, and yelled at the bear in an attempt to scare the animal away. The bear scampered into the woods.

Meanwhile, I sat on the picnic table trembling, adrenalin coursing through my veins. Although my dad told me to go and get my flip-flops, there was no way I would go back there. My oldest brother retrieved them for me. A bear totem[1], at age twelve, became a protective ally later in my life.

According to author Ted Andrews, in his book, *Animal Speak*, a totem is any natural object, being, or animal whose phenomena and energy we feel closely associated with during our life. Native American tradition teaches us animal totems are part of the human experience. It is in the interaction between humans and wildlife that an animal becomes a guide for the human. For example, when we see the same bird or wild animal come into our reality and associate it with a particular goodness or joyful event, that life form becomes our totem.

The first book of this two-part autobiography, *Enclosure: A Spiritual Autobiography*, ended in 2012. I've included more information and experiences of 2012 in this sequel.

---

1   A totem is a spirit being, sacred object, or symbol of a tribe, clan, family or individual. Some Native American tribe's tradition provides that each person is connected with nine different animals that will accompany him or her through life, acting as guides: https://www.legendsofamerica.com/na-totems/

CHAPTER 1

Leaving My Family
& Corporate Job

IT WAS THANKSGIVING DAY IN 2012, and my mother was not in a good mood. She announced, "I'm sick of it!" Something was different at this dinner, and my curiosity was piqued. There was small talk, nothing substantial, nor was anyone concerned about my current adventures. This would be the last Thanksgiving dinner my mother prepared for the family.

After dinner, I took my boyfriend, Peter, outside and told him from my inner knowing, "This is the last Thanksgiving meal we will attend with my family. I know this in my heart."

My shock had to be shared. I couldn't hold this realization in my consciousness by myself. Peter understood about shocking realizations because when his mother died, his father hadn't been able to manage caring for the four children and working full time on the Swiss railroad. Peter and his three siblings were placed in a Swiss orphanage. He'd experienced the ultimate abandonment of both parents.

I did not share with my family that my autobiography was written and about to be published. It would be my heartfelt surprise for them. It had taken ten months to prepare the manuscript and polish it with the expertise of the editors. After receiving the third edit, Shaman Lance advised me to book an appointment with Dr. Peebles regarding the preparation for publication. I felt the book was ready; however, I still had an ounce of doubt. When I considered that it was Dr. Peebles who held my completed book in his hand in a fellow participant's vision at the World Angel Day conference cohosted by Ann Albers and Jenny Cohen back in 2002, maybe Dr. Peebles was the more qualified to give me that answer. Surely, he would know if my book was ready to be published because he was in spirit and could see more than I could as a human.

I scheduled a private session with the famous trance channel, Summer Bacon, who channels Dr. Peebles for clients and groups. The date was September 10, 2012. Dr. Peebles, in his familiar Scottish accent, said to me, "God bless you indeed. Yes, it is. You are absolutely correct. There's no more that you can do. That would be like beating a dead horse, you see, and you want to keep it a live horse, yah?"

I replied, "Exactly. Thank you!"

Then I took this opportunity to confirm with Dr. Peebles of my channeling of Elizabeth Kuester, the Reiki master, and Jin Shin Jyutsu, a practitioner, for the introduction in *Enclosure: A Spiritual Autobiography.*

Dr. Peebles said, "Yah, and she says you did a 100 percent accurate job. She says, 'It's fabulous.' And she says she didn't so much express me through you. I just simply put an impression upon your heart, and you were actually able to write about it. And she says, 'I love your book. It's a beautiful, special gift to the world.' And she says, 'Really, I'm truly very honored to be a part of it.' "

I responded with tears, "I love her so much!"

Dr. Peebles added, "Yah, she loves you too. She says, 'I'm so proud of you. I wish I could be there [in the physical realm].' She says you could not have done this ten years ago. She says you were too scared. She says, 'Now, you're really going for it. You're just telling the world just like it is, and you're not trying to make anybody believe anything. You're not trying to force opinions on anybody. You're just saying, "Hey, here is what I believe. Here is what works for me." She says, 'You're not disguising it anymore.' She's so proud of you because you gave a dissertation that was very honest. It was rooted in integrity and human values. There are no mistakes in the world. You are embracing all of life. She loves that."

This was the confirmation I had been looking for. I felt much better and ready to push the "publish" button.

It was Monday, November 26, 2012, when my book, *Enclosure: A Spiritual Autobiography,* was finally published. Peter and I shared a bottle of cabernet sauvignon to celebrate. It had been a wonderful ten-month journey of preparing that book for publication.

I had left the corporate world for the last time. That was a mystical experience in itself, and I wrote about it in Enclosure. There was more to the story. I had been guided to seek a health review with an intuitive naturopathic doctor. This guidance came through a license plate that read, "NMD"—combined with a sign on the side of a utility repair truck that read, "Call Now." Through a recommendation by Lisa Montgomery, my feng shui consultant, Valeria Breiten, NMD, RD became my physician of choice. Her office style was one of calmness and peace. Dr. Breiten recommended a natural thyroid supplement for me because my thyroid was in overdrive from all the stress of working in a toxic environment with computers, electromagnetic frequencies, and the high productivity demands of reviewing medical claims. Sitting at a desk all day long didn't help either. Although I took my morning break on a patch of grass and did tai chi and qi gong, it wasn't enough. I rented a three-story apartment at the beginning of the year to give myself extra exercise up and down the double staircase and to live closer to the workplace. I began giving Angel Tarot Card readings in my apartment on the weekends. After one particular reading for a coworker, I sat down and looked at my bank account. Realizing I had enough money saved up to pay all my bills and transition to another place to rent, I went upstairs to my desk and wrote a heartfelt resignation letter.

Next was the matter of when I would submit my resignation. I asked for guidance and received it almost instantly. Looking at the thyroid supplement container, I noted it to be Thyroidinium 9CH. I had written it on the instruction sheet from Dr. Breiten and posted it on my refrigerator door. When it came time to reorder the preparation from the office, the receptionist said there was no 9CH. I thought, *Why would I write it down incorrectly?* When the correct bottle of thyroid supplement pellets came in the mail, sure enough, it wasn't 9CH. It was Thyroidinium 30C. There did exist a formulation called Thyroidinium 9CH, but it wasn't the prescription for me.

Messaging from our guides and angels can be fleeting and very subtle.

I began receiving more messages about when to leave this job, echoing the 9CH. I saw license plates that read 9CH. I wanted to give a two-week notice, and if I turned in my resignation the upcoming Friday, two weeks later would have been September 28, 2012.

Ordinarily, this date wouldn't mean much to most people; however, it was significant for me. Back in 2003, this was the date when I'd quit my job at an insurance company while I was married to my husband, Hoyt. He had been in Switzerland on a business trip. On September 28, 2007, I'd quit my job at another healthcare insurance company. And I'd met my current Swiss boyfriend, Peter, on September 28, 2008, in traffic school. As I had written in the first book, my deceased cat, Galileo, visited Peter and me in Switzerland at the end of summer vacation on September 28, 2009, one week before our return to the US.

I perceived this as a repeating sign and message that this would be the day to leave this company too. You may be asking what the significance was of the 9CH. The ninth month of the year was September. The Celtic tribe settling in that area were known as Helvetians, so the original name of Switzerland was *Confederatio Helvetica*, which is abbreviated as CH. I understood this message as when to leave the corporate job. Now, I had the time to develop my spiritual business.

For the remainder of 2012, I poured my energies into forming a public presence for Barbara Becker Healing. Guided by my Higher Self, I found a business mentor, MarVeena Meek[2], of Texas. While perusing the internet for a breathing meditation, I stumbled upon one of her instructional videos, then intuitively decided to check out her website. I looked at the landing page briefly, then clicked on the back button of my browser. The same landing page returned. I tried several more times, but it returned to her website! I knew someone was trying to get my attention, telling me to look further. This was when I discov-

---

2   https://www.marveena.com/

ered MarVeena offered a one-year business mentorship for those who wanted to take their spiritual services to the next level. She included a course on the tarot. This was exactly what I'd been searching for.

MarVeena had been a trick rider in her younger days. At age twenty-one, during a horse show, an accident occurred where the horse fell on top of her, causing severe injuries. The injuries were so life-threatening that she left her body and crossed over. Angels were surprised she'd shown up on the other side, and she was told to return to Earth. She was slammed back into her physical body and returned to the pain of her injuries. During her hospitalization, her clairvoyant psychic skills were opened. She began predicting people showing up to visit her in the hospital room, and her family members were stunned as each prediction came true within minutes of her foretelling. After MarVeena finished recovering at home, she became a standup comic. While sequentially reading books in the local library's metaphysical section, she stumbled upon the paranormal and psychic subjects. The rest was history, as she blossomed further and began giving tarot card readings, teaching spiritual business practices and procedures, and more.

My interest in learning the tarot had recently opened up. I had a deep-seated fear and resistance of the tarot from my Catholic upbringing and conditioning through books, movies, and religion. I wanted to face this fear once and for all. I wanted to know the truth. Tarot was the devil's work, wasn't it? I feared the subject due to my ignorance. Although I didn't mind that other psychic mediums used tarot cards to pass on messages for their clients, I felt it just wasn't for me, until now, in 2012.

I entered MarVeena's apprenticeship by writing a soul contract and signing it. The soul contract was written to establish everything I wanted to accomplish over the next year. After MarVeena gave me several suggestions for tarot card decks, I purchased the Alister Crowley Thoth Tarot Card deck and learned the traditional tarot through MarVeena's instructional videos and meditating with the cards. Can you imagine the look on my face when I discovered the tarot was the manual of how to be human? This was the manual I had been looking for my whole life! The tarot was about our spiritual journey on Earth through our human experience. Messages from the Higher Power come through the tarot and guide us in our everyday activities and expressions. In addition, the tarot helps us to understand our major life experiences like marriage, having children, accomplishments, and so much more. I didn't find one ounce of negativity or black magic involved! I had been misinformed. I made peace with this knowledge and my ignorance, knowing I could turn challenging messages into positive ones through messages from the angels.

MarVeena connected me with Rose Mis[3], a virtual assistant in New York City, to create a website for Barbara Becker Healing. Rose created an elegant website for me and taught me how to navigate and use it. She was thorough, professional, and competent in her work.

I wrote ten blog articles to get the blog up and running. Information was flowing out of me like a dam had broken upstream. I had so much to share from my earthly experiences, and it felt good to purge the challenges and apply the insights and wisdom I'd gained walking through them. Social media was a new concept for me. I had to learn how to make friends on Facebook, which was daunting. Sitting on the staircase in my apartment with my head in my hands, I said to myself, "I don't know how to make friends!" I sounded utterly ridiculous because I could make friends in life, but this was different. I asked my angels for help. And then MarVeena helped me approach people on social media with integrity and truth.

I kept all my posts on social media positive, uplifting, and geared toward helping humanity. Sometimes my posts were humorous. Sometimes they were about a worthy cause, such as helping children, animals, or promoting other's service to humanity based in the heart. Occasionally, I would post a controversial topic or video for us to consider. For me, social media was one marketing tool to help people find me, my books, and my services, and a way to connect with people, listen to the pulse of the global mind, and offer positive perspectives for others to reflect upon. Social media could also be a dark place with disinformation, misinformation, and victim mentality. This was where we lightworkers planted our truth and light to uplift others.

Back in 2004, I used the Doreen Virtue Angel Healing cards to

---

3   https://www.rosemis.com/

convey messages for my clients. Doreen considered these cards to be "beginner" cards for her students. After I learned the tarot, Doreen Virtue and professional intuitive, Radleigh Valentine, published their collaborative project of the Angel Tarot Card[4] deck in 2012. When I saw the card's artwork by Stephen A. Roberts, I instantly fell in love with the soft, gentle, beautiful colored images depicting angels, fairies, merpeople, dolphins, whales, and unicorns. I knew I wanted to convey messages for my clients with a deck like this, so I took their online course for Angel Tarot Card Reading in December of 2012. When I practiced with other students online, the recipients of my readings enjoyed the readings and resonated with the messages I channeled for them. I felt encouraged to enroll in the Advanced Angel Tarot Card Reading online course in 2013 to give me further insight into the meanings of the cards. I soon incorporated the tarot into my angel readings for clients.

I began the journey of book promotion by researching the venues and finding it does cost money to promote your work. I knew I would be supported. It was just a matter of time. My book was available as an eBook and a paperback at all of the major online retailers. I was grateful to receive monthly royalty payments. Everyone I knew and met congratulated me for publishing my autobiography. Well, almost everyone.

I presented my book to my parents on December 30, 2012, while announcing my entrepreneurship of Barbara Becker Healing, LLC, in the living room of their home. I wasn't expecting their accolades; however, it would have been nice to receive a smidgeon of support. That was not the case. They refused to believe that I could have a service to humanity and support myself. The first thing my mother asked was about how my automobile was running. I replied that my SUV recently received a green light inspection with new tires and good brakes. The message from her was about fear. I just couldn't accept it. She refused to believe that I channeled healing energies for people. When I shared with her that there are medical doctors who understand energetic healing and my channeling gift, she still refused to believe it. I said to her,

---

4   https://radleighvalentine.com/shop/angel/ Please note Doreen Virtue was no longer associated with tarot cards or angels as of 2017.

"Okay, let's agree to disagree." Being right isn't important anymore to me. Loving allowance for her to have her opinion was conducive in the grand scheme of consciousness and relationships. My father sat in his living room recliner, refusing to talk or look at me. It was time for me to leave.

As I walked toward the front door, I received an inner knowing message. *"This will be the last time you see your parents alive."* It felt like I was walking in slow motion, in a dreamlike state. Part of my mind didn't want to accept this knowledge, and the other part understood. When I drove down the road and back to my apartment, I realized that my parents were the only ones who did not share my good news of becoming a published author. It would be several more years when I received information about what was occurring regarding this interaction with my parents.

It was time for me to move.

My apartment lease ended at the beginning of 2013. I moved to a five-bedroom home I rented across town in Tempe, Arizona, where I offered channeled healing sessions and angel tarot card readings. This meant my travel to the ranch in Wickenburg to be with Peter every other weekend would be longer, but he had placed the ranch on the market and was already holding open house tours in the hopes of selling the property so we could downsize to a shared townhome in Wickenburg.

On one such weekend, during an open house at the Sombrero ranch, I was in my bedroom on the other side of the house when a woman came to look through the house. I was unaware anyone had come to walk through as I sat at my desk in the middle of the room, typing on my computer. I heard someone in the hallway, just outside my bedroom door, and gave a disgusted sigh. I didn't hear footsteps on the concrete floor of the hallway, nor did anyone enter the bedroom.

Later, Peter told me a woman had come to walk through the house. He'd told her she could wander down the hall and go into each of the four bedrooms, and his girlfriend was in the last bedroom and could answer questions. When the woman returned to the living room where Peter sat on the sofa, she was disappointed that when she went into the last bedroom, I was not there. Even though I was sitting in a chair in the middle of the room, she could not see me when she entered the room!

This was an example of me vibrating in the fifth dimension, and the woman was vibrating in the third dimension. She was not a happy person to begin with because Peter said she made derogatory comments about the house as soon as she walked in. I found it fascinating that I could hear her sigh but not see her either.

When I moved into the Tempe home, I hired feng shui master, consultant, and teacher, Lisa Montgomery. I'd known her for years. Lisa and her husband, Charles, owned and operated Feng Shui AZ[5], a store and education center, to inform the public and feng shui practitioners about the art of establishing the correct flow of energy in a person's home, office, or business. Feng shui, which means "wind-water," iss the Chinese practice of looking at our environments and how we live in harmony with the principles of the natural world, including energy movement. She'd prepared the energy flow in the three-story apartment I rented in 2012. We prepared the Tempe home for the optimal energy flow and a blessing for all to prosper in good health. In the Chinese astrology reading she gave me, she said the summer months would be a good time to be conservative with money management and that in the fall, the money flow would certainly increase.

In addition to the energy flow adjustment, I felt it was time to receive a healing session with Grandma Chandra in Mesa, Arizona. This would be my first private session with Gma, as she was called. Grandma Chandra is the daughter of Cat Parenti. Born in a physically challenged body, Gma saw only with her third eye. She couldn't talk, but she was able to make sounds through her vocal cords. She used a walker to stabilize her gait. From my perspective, Gma was far from challenged. She was an amazing, beautiful, ascended master from a White planet with a joyful sense of humor. She is very brilliant and could facilitate healing for others. Gma had taught her mother mental telepathy, and this was one of the ways she communicated. Her mother, Cat, was an angel. Gma's father was a Sufi Master who was killed in the Afghanistan war. If you would like to know more about Cat and

---

5   http://www.southwesternfengshui.com/

Gma, I recommend you read Cat's two-volume books, *Afghanistan: From Kabul to Brooklyn.*[6]

I received a one-hour guided meditation remotely in the house with Grandma. She was in the living room, and I was seated in her home office in a chair. I was bathed in a magenta color light from a light source across the room. Listening to dolphin songs, I saw all sorts of animals, dolphins, and whales through my third eye. When I returned from the altered state of consciousness, Cat helped to ground me by reciting a beautiful grounding meditation mantra.

I walked out to the living room and sat on one of the two sofas, and Grandma and Cat sat on the other. The "reading" began, where Gma told me information and answered questions. Grandma said I am a whale, just like her. We were brothers at the time that Jesus walked the Earth. We were part of his entourage, not his disciples. She confirmed that I'm a Zagian, and my planet is outside our solar system, very far away in another star system. She was a little surprised when she realized my energy vibration matched hers.

Suddenly, Gma raised herself up from the sofa, walked over to me with her walker, and laid down on the sofa with her head buried in the right side of my abdomen. Cat instructed me to take off my eyeglasses. When I placed them on the side table, I slipped into an altered state of consciousness. I vaguely remember singing tones and chanting. Cat noticed that Gma and I were holding hands during this healing. "Gma doesn't hold hands with anyone!" Cat told me later. This was a first!

Gma said I was a captured slave during the Roman times and had a collar with a chain, which was the basis of my throat chakra problem that we were addressing now. Many lightworkers who have problems with their throat chakras have been enslaved, tortured, and murdered for their gifts. Their mortal wound involved the throat area. The cellular memories from our previous lives were still in our bodies until we released them. Gma prescribed oils for fear and love. One drop of each to my third eye (forehead) every night until gone. I felt a shift within me after the healing. It was a humbling honor to receive a healing session with Gma and Cat.

---

6   Parenti, Cat. *Afghanistan: A Memoir From Brooklyn to Kabul* (books 1 and 2). Forchianna Publishing, 2019.

On February 4, 2013, I participated in a group blessing ceremony with Lisa Montgomery outside her feng shui store in Scottsdale, Arizona. This ceremony was performed on the first new moon of the year, also known as the Chinese New Year. People set their intentions for what they want to accomplish and resolve in the year to come. Intentions included abundance in health and wealth, good relationships, prosperous careers, and harmony and balance in all aspects of life. It was like participating in a birthday party without the cake. Everyone was happy and positive.

During the Chinese New Year ceremony, we hold oranges with small red candles inserted into the top of the fruit. Our intentions for the year to come were spoken in unison out loud, facing the four directions.

On the same night of the Chinese New Year Festival, I met the delightful owner of a store that specialized in angel decorations, cards, wind chimes, etc. She invited me to give angel readings at her store during the Parada Del Sol (Parade of the Sun) celebration for a couple of hours and was also looking for an angel communicator to do readings once a week.

On Wednesday of that same week, before I drove up to the Sombrero Ranch home, I felt an urgency for urination. It disappeared quickly, and I didn't give it another thought. I prepared a wonderful breakfast with Peter. The house felt so warm and cozy with the smell of cooked eggs, hazelnut coffee, English muffins, and assorted fruits with yogurt. My heart was so happy and filled with high energy. I worked on my first newsletter and sent the test version to my virtual assistant.

The night before the Parada Del Sol angel reading event, I experienced urgency again, plus the burning and frequency of urination. My urine was cloudy and dark blood red. I went to the nearest pharmacy and bought an over-the-counter bladder pain remedy. The first pill worked, but the second one did not. The next day, I texted my naturopathic physician. She texted back with instructions to go to a natural grocery store that offers homeopathic remedies. I bought D-mannose, Staphysagria 30C, and a bottle of undiluted cranberry juice. D-mannose was a simple sugar naturally found in foods and supplements we eat, used to prevent and treat urinary tract infections. The cranberry juice produced an alkaline environment that inhibits the growth of bacteria in our bladders. The Staphysagria was used to relieve pain.

I went to the Angel Store early the next morning and began setting up my table outside the shop. The temperature outside was in the forties, and the wind was blowing hard. I bundled up with my black leather gloves, down jacket, and cashmere scarf. It was cold for this desert dweller! I tried my best not to think of the uncomfortable sensations nagging at me in my bladder and prayed my angels would help me be as comfortable as possible. I smiled the whole three hours and telepathically told people to go into the Angel Store. It was fun watching people walk by, stop, and turn around and go into the store. At noon, the store owner stepped outside to tell me it was a good day for her. I was happy for her prosperity.

I had a premonition in the morning that an old friend and fellow energy worker, Carol, would show up, and she did. She graciously bought my book and purchased an angel reading. She really didn't need one. The reading was confirmation of what she already knew. She was an amazing healer in her own right. However, confirmation readings can be the most enjoyable for a client and are fun for me. It always feels good when we know we're right on track with our soul path. She was well, and her horizons were expanding. I was so happy for her and wished her the best. I left the store at 12:30 p.m., and Carol graciously helped me load up my car. I found out later there were two more requests for angel readings after I had already left town.

The Angel Store owner called the next day and asked if I would perform weekly angel readings. I agreed and returned on that Friday. She was surprised I came. She was used to angel readers not being on time or not showing up at all. The first Friday of readings was delightful. I felt very happy to do three angel readings for customers. Each person left filled with inspiration and clarity in the questions they asked.

The following week, I went to my homeopathic physician's office. We talked for two hours, trying to get to the reason for my urinary tract symptoms. The preparations she'd prescribed the prior week had helped immensely. She tested my urine and found a large number of leukocytes indicating an infection; however, my angels told me I was inflamed, not infected. The physician was perplexed about the root cause of my symptoms. She then asked, "Tell me what was going on in your life."

I shared with her that my parents, to this day, had not acknowledged an ounce of support for the work of writing and publishing my autobiography. There was not a gleam of happiness when I handed them copies of my book. In fact, when I shared that I no longer worked in the corporate environment and instead had a business as a full-time angel communicator and healing channel, my mother had replied, "You're a failure!" I told the physician that the last time I called my mother, she said she didn't want to talk with me if I said anything about my spiritual healing work and activities. My response to my mother before I hung up the phone was, "As you wish."

In response to this information, Dr. Breiten said, "Barbara, if my family treated me the way your family treats you, I'd be very angry."

I looked at her and replied, "Of course! I'm pissed!"

Light bulbs lit up above our heads. This revelation brought me comfort. Now that I had my truth in front of me, I had to get into the feeling of anger so I could process it. As Dr. Breiten advised, I placed white light around each member of my family and a black obsidian shield around me, so I would not feel the lower vibration energy. I stopped all contact with my family. After two weeks, all symptoms were gone.

Dr. Breiten gave me more advice regarding this interpersonal relationship change. I had to come up with a sign or symbol that I would know a family member had had a change of heart and would contact me to reconnect. I shared with her that I could feel vibrations in email messages, the written word, voice mail messages, and the words a person used in their oral communications. She also shared with me that if a family member has a death bed request for me to visit one last time, I am obligated to do so. I agreed with this concept. Other than that, I was to stay away from my family for the sake of my health. I knew this was serious. Someone was giving me a message. It was me, my Higher Self. In my book, *Time Travels: Exploration of Lives Remembered*, I revealed who my Higher Self is. We (because we are not separate from our Higher Self) are a collective of beings from the Great Central Sun of 10,000 suns. All loving, all correcting, all balancing, frequency, consciousness, entities, planets, stars, all the power that emanates from the Great Central Sun comprises the thousands of my Higher Self. I have come to learn over the years that they also are composed of physicians of all disciplines and specialties. They have the ability to do surgery on my clients during healing sessions, and the client no longer has pain nor ailment. If I didn't pay attention and take action, then I would receive the proverbial two-by-four upside the head, often expressed in a terminal illness, such as cancer. My survival was dependent upon my separation from my family.

One of my family members left a voice message that the family felt I belonged in a straightjacket and locked up in a mental institution because I talk with angels and dead people. For several days, I pondered this decision not to have any communication with my family. I loved them very much and was torn between standing up for myself and wanting to honor and respect my family. I believe in the concept of a family loving and supporting one another. Embracing and expressing joy when a member accomplishes goals and projects is what families were supposed to do. I just couldn't understand why my family would not support me and allow me to be who I am.

Still, there was a nagging doubt about if I was taking the right action. I'd worked so hard on loving myself and finding love in others. What was I missing? What was I not comprehending? There was someone who could help me put this into perspective—my tai chi instructor, a member of the Table of Ancients and spiritual guide for humanity, Grandmaster Zeysan. If he counseled other people, certainly his counsel could help me.

I called Zeysan and told him about my latest life challenge. I called him because I wanted to make sure I'd covered all bases and saw the situation clearly. His words gave me confirmation, comfort, and a clearer perspective.

He said, "Well, Barb, you're finally taking your power back. Your family has been sucking your power your entire life. Now that they have to stand in their own power, it's freaking them out, and they don't know what to do. You're going to have to stand up for yourself and speak your truth sometime."

I knew that, at least for now, there was no returning to my family. I was beginning to understand that they were giving me the ultimate gift of love, sacrificing themselves as the loving beings they are, for me to walk away and not look back. It was time for me to continue my journey and the work I'd agreed to do while incarnated as a human on Earth.

Although my family may not have understood their behavior and my lack of contact with them, here in the physical human form, I loved them even more. I knew they were playing roles for me to learn my lessons and walk my soul path. I knew in my heart that someday, hopefully soon, I would have a greater comprehension of this grand act of love they were engaged in for me. I was not the victim, but rather the experiencer who was grateful for everything. This perspective empowered me and rendered peace within me.

For some who are reading this, it may seem like Barbara has flipped her wig and has it all wrong. While I agree with you that my life has flipped, I saw this exact scenario playing out in other families. I began to receive Angel Tarot Card reading clients whose families had abandoned them on an emotional level. Family personalities were changing, and my clients were having a very hard time dealing with it. It was as if lightworkers were being thrown out of their families. I tried my best to explain the truth, but my clients were not prepared to deal with the pain of abandonment. The victimhood programs are still running. As long as a person thinks they are a victim, they won't be able to process and heal their wounds.

I debated in my mind about writing about this major life experience in this book. I knew I had to because it may shed some light for someone else going through similar circumstances. Stay with me, dear reader, because later, I will reveal more going on behind the scenes.

Much more.

CHAPTER 2

Creating the
Star Energy Healing Group

A FTER SHARING MY HEALING ABILITIES with Dr. Breiten, she recommended I read Paramhansa Yogananda's *Autobiography of a Yogi*. The book nearly fell in my lap when a friend and fellow tai chi student, Roy, gifted me with his copy. Roy was downsizing his library and graciously let me choose some books to keep.

I devoted an hour each morning to reading the yoga master's biography. His life story and the lessons he learned stirred a resonance within me from the voice of his written words. I became intrigued with the form of yoga he'd brought to the Western world back in the 1950s, called Kriya Yoga[7]. I searched the internet for a local Kriya Yoga course and found a nearby center where people gathered weekly to perform Kriya Yoga in a sacred space. I contacted the leader of the center and made arrangements to attend the informational presentation with a traveling instructor scheduled to come to the Phoenix area. Subsequently, I applied for the Kriya Yoga initiation course to be held on the first weekend of April.

In March of 2013, I received a message through a social media platform from a woman who told me she was about to commit suicide. She'd found my website and purchased *Enclosure: A Spiritual Autobiography*. By the time she finished reading the book, she no longer had a desire to end her life. She'd contacted me to tell her story. After our conversation, I sat in my office and cried tears of gratitude for my courage to share my life story, recalling how my ego had protested while I was writing the book, telling me I couldn't write those experiences. What if I hadn't put them in? If I'd left my experiences out of the story, would the book have had enough impact on someone who was feeling so depressed and hopeless? This woman was confirmation that I had made the best decision. For her, I'm eternally grateful.

I received my Kriya Yoga attunement on April 6, 2013. I signed a nondisclosure agreement, which prevents me from sharing the details of the weekend activities. What I can share was the beautiful sensation I felt flowing into my body from the crown chakra downward during the ceremony. Tears of joy ran down my cheeks at that moment.

On the 14th of April, Peter and I left Wickenburg for a short vacation on the west coast of the US. He needed to go to the Swiss Embassy in Los Angeles to renew his Swiss passport. The husband of my best friend from childhood, Dianne, died on April 17, 2013, after a four-year, courageous battle with cancer. They had been married for thirty-three years. Over the years, Dianne and I had communicated at least once a year by phone. As we'd dived deeper into our life experiences, there grew a separation. It had been several years since we'd talked.

On May 10, 2013, I received a message from my angels. "Barbara, it's time to start the group healings again." They were referring back to 2004 when I was asked to come to small groups of people, channeling the healing energies while I was still receiving the downloads and energetic changes in my body and energy fields. I wrote about these experiences in chapter seven of my first book, *Enclosure: A Spiritual Autobiography*.

My friend, Cansu, recommended I look into the meetup.com platform on the internet to organize a gathering. I asked my angels what to call this group healing event. They replied, "Star Energy Healing Group." I sent out a message for those interested in this form of healing to meet me at the Pomegranate restaurant in Chandler, Arizona, on Friday, the 24th of May. There, I introduced myself as a star being and told them about my gifts of the mathematical star language and my psychic skills. As a gift for coming to lunch and meeting others of like mind, I gave mini-angel readings at the table. Ten people came. I asked a dear friend who channeled the angels while playing her Omnichord to play music during the channeling. The angels took over her body as she surrendered, and the music was heavenly and healing. At the time, I had known Barbara South for more than five years. I was a guest for a brief period of time, giving angel readings and transmitting the healing energies on her internet radio show back in 2008. After receiving the "Heart's Desire Blessing" and a sacred rose oil anointing from a Buddhist monk, she began creating beautiful spontaneous music with the channeled angels in her body. Barbara came to the introduction lunch too.

Fifteen people came to the first Star Energy Healing group gathering, held at the office of referral expert, Sandy Rogers, in downtown Phoenix, Arizona, on April 29, 2013. I helped everyone relax into a meditative state through a visualization technique. As Barbara South and the angels played music, I surrendered into an altered state of consciousness. My body walked around the room while "they" moved my hands and arms in gesticulated patterns. When I returned to the seat at the front of the group, I was guided to speak the mathematical star language. After the transmission, angelic tones sang from my vocal cords. And then, it was complete. I guided everyone to return to their bodies and become grounded.

In sharing their experiences, one woman said her nephew, who had crossed over, came and spoke with her, which was very healing for her. She had tears when she hugged me at the end of the gathering. Another woman felt a "procedure" with instruments occurring in her neck for her cervical pain, and she felt much better afterward. People saw angels and fairies in the room. What was more intriguing to me, though, was what happened to Sandy, sitting at her office desk in the next room. Although there was a brick wall between the two rooms, Sandy said that all of a sudden, she felt vibrations in her body. She surrendered to the healing. They were working on her too, through a brick wall! This was the first time I was aware that people nearby received the healing energy too. It would not be the last.

On May 14, 2013, I went to a Braco[8] live gazing event at the Crescent Sheraton Hotel in Phoenix, Arizona. Braco, in the form of golden light, came to me the day before at two o'clock in the morning, in my bedroom, and invited me to come and assist the many rather than the few. My dear friend, Ann Albers, attended these gazing events also. Ann's presence made the experience much more special for me. Anyone who knows Ann can feel the energy and light rise in a room just from her very presence. After each gazing by Braco, the support team asked for testimonials. This meant we had to walk up to the front of the audience and speak before three live streaming television cameras. When I volunteered and walked toward the front, I heard Ann squeal with delight that I would participate in the joy while sharing my experience.

During the gaze, I could see beams of golden light shining down from the high ballroom ceiling into each person's head. And because I can see into the dimensions, I also saw our dear extraterrestrial friends in the cosmos, in their spacecrafts, saying to me that they could feel the love and healing emanating from this gathering of beautiful souls, sharing and receiving the love from God, Source Creator. It was revealed to me that what was being created there in that room was being felt throughout the universe! I also felt a physical sensation of pressure behind my left eye during the gaze because I had asked for my eyesight to return to 20/20 vision, or at least better vision.

Also interesting for me was that the whole day felt like a square dance, with changing partners, as I connected with many people. When I ran out of business cards, I retrieved more from my car. A man asked me to be interviewed on his radio show. People came and thanked me for what I'd said before the audience. I accepted whatever God wanted me to do and where to be, just following my soul as to where to sit in the ballroom. I noticed several people insisted on sitting next to me, and I just witnessed their healing energy during the gazing. People came up to me and shared their recommendations of various healing exercises for my eye vision. I took the advice into consideration.

On May 22, 2013, I received an attunement while lying on my bed.

8   https://www.braco.me/en/

My Higher Self told me to lay down and that one was coming. The energies traveled through my body at lightning speed for about ten seconds. I had fallen down that morning on the living room tile floor, and my left thigh felt sore. After going to the park and doing qi gong and tai chi, I felt much lighter, as if in a new, lighter version of my body, if that was possible.

On June 7, 2013, I facilitated another Star Energy Healing Group in Gilbert, Arizona, then kept searching for another venue to hold the healing groups. Two weeks later, on June 21, the Star Energy Healing Group met at a healing place called Angel Wings Wellness Center. I met Debbie, who was co-owner of the business through a man I'd sat next to at lunch at the Pomegranate Cafe in Chandler, Arizona, the week before. I'd told him I was looking for another venue for the gatherings, and he'd suggested Angel Wings. Angel Wings Wellness Center had a room for yoga and meditation. The size of the room was perfect for my small groups. Debbie provided relaxing aromatherapy, cleared the energy of the room, and arranged the chairs prior to our events. Participants shared their healing experiences after the energy transmissions, like dental pain stopping, worry and anxiety feelings dissolved, and feeling inspired and at peace. These one-hour sessions ended at 7:00 p.m., but no one wanted to leave. People felt "blissed-out."

The radio show producer I'd met at the Braco event in May asked me to be a psychic on his radio show. However, he had to vet me through an angel reading. I gave him a reading over the phone. He said I was the real deal because I picked up on attributes no one else knew about him. He arranged for a venue in Sedona for me to channel the healing energies for the public. The venue he found, however, was closed down due to a mold infestation. Repairs had to be done before business operations could resume. This information was given to me only the week before the planned event. The woman who owned the closed venue gave me several other places to check out. The producer was out of town, so this was left to me to arrange. I called the first name on the list, Creative Life Center of Sedona[9], and booked a room. The week before the event, the producer was able to return to Sedona and change all of the flyers on bulletin boards in town.

---

9   https://www.sedonacreativelife.com/

A small group of people came to the Sedona Room at the Creative Life Center for my Star Energy Healing group event. Barbara South came with me to provide the angelic music. Before the evening event began, a blonde woman and a brunette woman came and sat in chairs in the middle of the room. The blonde woman approached me and said, "Barbara, my friend I came with never goes to any group events in Sedona. However, when she saw your photo on the flyer at the grocery store bulletin board, she emphatically stated, 'I must see her!' " I told the blonde woman, "Thank you for letting me know."

I told the group to close their eyes and prepare for relaxation. As the music began, I allowed my Higher Self to move my body. My arms swung in symbols through the air. I walked around the group and gave each person a unique experience by adjusting their star codes around their heads.

As I walked to the front of the room, I was guided to sit down in my chair and wait until the music stopped. Then I spoke the mathematical star language for about five minutes. Afterward, I guided everyone back into their bodies, channeled messages, and answered questions from the participants.

After the one-hour event, the brunette woman approached me and said, "Barbara, years ago, I was abducted and tortured on a spaceship. I worked on that trauma and released it. I help others who have similar experiences. When you began that star language, I saw all of the torture memories coming up again. In my head, I said to myself, *Oh no!* Barbara, suddenly, it all just melted away. You're doing good work. Keep it up!"

I thanked her for that significant confirmation.

The Star Energy Healing Groups continued through the summer at Angel Wings Wellness Center. I also continued working on myself through various modalities. Working with Grandmother Chandra was one of the ways I cleared my energy fields and assisted Mother Earth.

CHAPTER 3

Grandmother Chandra

GRANDMA CHANDRA WAS THE DAUGHTER of Cat Parenti and Sufi master Jamal Mahmoud Yusuf Khan. She received all of her father's gifts of bilocation, distance healing, saving those in perilous situations when it was not their time to die, and walking the soul out of the body when it is ready to transition back home to Source. She remembered all of her past lives. She was extremely brilliant in intellect and fulfilling her lifelong mission to raise planetary consciousness through codes and frequencies in her work using sacred geometry and quantum physics. If you would like to learn more about Grandma Chandra, I recommend reading her mother's two-book volume titled *Afghanistan: From Brooklyn to Kabul* and visit her website at: grandmachandra.com.

May 30, 2013, felt special. I'd received a free psychic reading for winning a contest given by Grandma Chandra to name her newsletter. I thought Grandma's Galactic Gazette sounded whimsical and appropriate for her. In a private chat with Grandma, I asked for the name of my home star planet. Telepathically through Cat, Gma said the planet's name was Loeluliy, pronounced *low-loo-lee*. Loeluliy is outside of our Earth's solar system, where I am a Zagian being. As I mentioned in my first book, Zagians are a culture of beings who are balanced in the feminine and masculine energies but not very emotional. I went to planet Earth to learn emotions and then teach them to the Zagians. My

Zagian ability to stay calm and centered had served me well during my years as a critical care and emergency room nurse.

On June 2, 2013, I was participating in Gma's galactic teleseminar. I can't share about the other participants; however, my throat chakra was worked on during this event. I felt intense energy coming into my crown chakra and down throughout my body. I saw myself traveling with great speed inside a wormhole. I then saw myself traveling over the ocean, becoming a whale, and seeing a woman drumming. A Native American spirit came into my vision. The woman opened a box, and I was given a purple Andara[10].

Andaras are a form of glass that enhances your creations, heart intentions, and dream state. In the United States, Andaras are found on land belonging to the family of Lady Neli, a Choctaw Medicine Woman who found the first one in February of 1967 on her property in Northern California. Andaras from this area are located with a white powdery substance that has a high frequency of monatomic atoms called Etherium. Etherium was used throughout history to raise a person's vibratory states and expand consciousness.

I stepped into the purple Andara and was given a peacock blue Andara. With my physical mouth wide open, through my third eye, I could see a blue light directed over my throat area.

During the debriefing, Grandma said I had received a major activation, and a past life healing was done for the past life where I had been punished for speaking my truth.

One thing I've noticed in a person's healing over the years was there are certain wounds that are received lifetime after lifetime. For some, several healing sessions or modalities are needed to remove the past life residue that causes their current life physical issues.

Three days later, Shaman Lance[11] dropped by the house in Tempe and gave me a throat chakra clearing in my home office. While sitting up in my desk chair, my body shook as Lance used my blue quartz pendant to activate the healing. Tones came forth from my throat, and I went into a brief altered state of consciousness from which I returned to being alert and awake. It was a lovely, gentle healing.

---

10   http://www.mickeymagic.com/healing/authentic_andaras.html
11   https://www.lanceheard.com/

On June 6, 2013, I gave a combination angel reading and healing transmission by phone for a young woman in the Midwest. Her fear and anxiety stemmed from a prior life as a white witch. She was powerful, and we were together in the same life in the mid-1700s. She was killed with a guillotine. She was remembering being sliced in half from something coming down on her. Her angel guide was helping her with her fear and anxiety and, now off work on medical leave from the toxic environment she worked in, she couldn't leave her apartment. The thought of leaving her apartment brought about severe anxiety. Her angels gave her affirmations for security, saying she needed to relax more, soak in lavender oil and sea salt baths, play for balance, and engage in more laughter, and she would see herself transcend this problem. Two days later, she texted me from a local park, feeling much better. Her life blossomed into a new career after the session, and she was no longer confined to the apartment, evidenced by her air travel to the other side of the world for training in a natural modality for healing and nourishment of people. It was an honor to have given this young woman a powerful healing session transmitted across the United States by phone.

On June 7, I facilitated the Star Energy Healing group event at a venue in Gilbert, Arizona, called Angel Wings Wellness Center. This was a large room with chairs, adjustable lighting, and aromatherapy fragrance to calm participants. It was fascinating for me to see people in a serene state of bliss at the end of the evening. One woman, in particular, noted her dental pain was gone as a result of the healing energies of the mathematical star language. On June 21, fifteen people came to the Star Energy Healing group at Angel Wings. These gatherings of healing were given twice a month at this calm and peaceful venue for the rest of the summer.

Later that summer, Lance called me with an important message. He was hesitant to tell me the dream he'd had the night before and that it involved Peter and me. I could tell from his hesitance that he felt very uncomfortable, concerned about my comfort and how I would receive the information, but I knew deep down I could handle anything he would say. I encouraged him to tell me and that I would easily place it on a shelf, so to speak, and ponder it later. With that permission, Lance told me that in his dream, Peter was unfaithful to me. Peter would have a new girlfriend and enter into a new relationship while we are together. He didn't know when this would happen, just that it would happen. I thanked Lance for this information; however, this was so far from Peter's principles that the likelihood of it coming to fruition would be one in a million. I understood that people could be blindsided and life's circumstances change, but what Lance described was so far from the philosophy about relationships that Peter shared with me, I considered it very unlikely. The bottom line was that I trusted Lance and knew he was giving me this information for a reason. What that reason was would need to be revealed down the road. I am grateful Lance trusted me enough to give me difficult information. My responsibility was to take the information into consideration and not "kill the messenger."

On June 15, as I drove on the Rio Salado Parkway in Mesa, Arizona, I stopped at the traffic light at the Loop 101 freeway. To my right was one of the Maricopa County Animal shelters. I heard the voice of a dog talk to me in plain English, saying, "Barbara, please come here."

I replied, "I will come as soon as I can." The feeling within me wasn't one of emergency but rather of great concern.

Two days later, I arrived at the shelter, walked in, and asked silently, *Now what?*

The voice said, "Keep going."

I entered one of the areas where there were long buildings of dogs in cages. This reminded me of a prison—a prison in hell. The flooring was bare concrete. There were no cushions or blankets to rest upon. Each dog had an area that was outdoors. Swamp coolers blew cool, moist air. The stench from the feces and urine was overwhelming, but I persevered because I had been asked to come. I intuitively began to walk to each cage and tell each dog that I love them. The mathematical star language was spoken. Some of the cages had four to five small dogs in them. There were dogs recovering from surgery, and I directed healing energy toward all of them. I went through four of these long corridors, then over to the cat and small animal area and expressed my love for them too. I blessed all the people working in this facility.

These were dogs that, for some reason, became strays or were given up because the family could no longer afford their care. When

I returned home, I called a woman who communicated with animals. She told me of someone working to change these types of shelters so the animals are given a more pleasant environment.

One such example was the Humane Society facility in Wickenburg, Arizona. I visited the facility and found a beautiful place for our furry friends. The cat room had cat trees, soft beds, toys, fresh food, and water. Symphonic music was played during the daytime. It was a clean environment with a doorway for the cats to walk outside to an enclosure for their safety and well-being, to breathe fresh air. There was a poster on the wall with photos of each cat, displaying their name and pertinent history. For the dogs, each had a clean holding area with access outdoors. The volunteers exercised the dogs daily. I was given a private introduction to each dog the first time I visited. My confirmation of the good care the volunteers were giving these dogs was when I returned the next month and saw most of the dog kennels were empty because they had been adopted. What a good feeling to know these fur babies had new homes!

On July 14, 2013, I participated in an intergalactic meditation with Gma. I saw the Eye of God nebula in outer space, then went to Hawaii and merged with Gma to become a whale. I was floating in seaweed. Codes were retrieved. I held onto a violet light tube torus twenty-four inches in diameter and directed it to various places on the planet, then out to the cosmos. Each time, I said mentally, *Light and love.* I received an intense download of energy.

Athena Star[12] (a psychic medium who assists Gma during the teleseminars) said, "You have an A++ for the work you have been doing!" This must have been in reference to my Kriya Yoga and loving God as much as possible. I strive for more each day. I believe the Kriya Yoga masters spoke through Athena. (*"Yes, yes, yes,"* Grandma Chandra said in my mind).

The next morning, I woke up and noticed my face no longer had the blemishes I'd been treating for the past two years. The right side was less red. I made an appointment with Debbie, a hypnotherapist, to explore hypnosis, releasing my blocks and resistance to a deeper surrender and increased vulnerability for me to continue to trance

12   https://www.athenastar.com/

channel. I firmly resolved to ask God to take away and place in the fire all thoughts and feelings of anger, evil, pride, viciousness, insincerity, suspicion, doubt, envy, jealousy, greed, control over another, etc. I began focusing and perceiving that God was doing everything. God breathes. God lives. I am consciousness, and God has given me this beautiful body and breath so that I can live and reach Self Realization—a human's life reincarnation goal. I'm in this graduate school of spirituality with a determination and intention to become self-realized, if it's possible in this lifetime.

As the renter of this five-bedroom home in Tempe, I was also the steward of a sacred Navajo painting located on a wall in the living room. This acrylic painting was quite large, at eight feet wide and four feet in height. I was told the Navajo artist had been required to receive permission from the elders to even paint the picture. I was guessing the reason was that the painting had seven supernatural spirits in it, known as the Yeibichai[13]. I imagined the elders looked into the future to see who would be in stewardship of this painting, saw me, and knew that I would respect the spirits, the energy, and the healing properties of this work of art and soul. I could feel the powerful energy emanating from this painting and enjoyed sitting in meditation with it. I felt at home in the energies.

One day, I spoke with the spirits of the painting and told them I had a question. I also told them I would abide by whatever answer they gave me. Honoring them and their counsel was of utmost importance to me because I respected them. I asked, "Could I have permission to take a photograph of the painting. I promise not to post the photo on social media or in a blog."

The answer was, "No."

I responded, "Very well. Thank you."

A female participant from the Star Energy Healing Group came to the Tempe house for a healing session. In my healing sessions, I helped the client to relax into a deep state of sleep using sound and the energy from Source flowing through my hands. The client laid on a Reiki (or

---

13   It is said the Yeibichai are supernatural beings who created the Navajo people and taught them how to live in harmony with the universe. Upon request from a medicine man, the Yeibichai have the power to heal someone.

massage) table with a blanket for comfort. The room was darkened with drapes on the window. I had a white tea light candle lit for ambient light. I received instruction in my mind from my guides for where to place my hands over the client's body and when to adjust the star codes above their body. After the energy session was complete, I sat in a chair and quietly waited for the client to return to consciousness.

What happened in this healing session was different from any other I had ever facilitated. When I sat down, I saw the Yeibichai enter the room through the closed closet doors, dancing around the client in a line. They made just one pass around the table, then danced back through the closet doors. I watched this with my eyes wide open and then thanked the Yeibichai for participating in the healing of my client.

In this particular client, her main issue was childhood trauma of being raped by a family member. What she hadn't told me before the session was that her left knee was swollen and painful. During the session, my guides told me to place my hands around her left knee, about two to three inches from the surface. When she returned the next month, she told me her knee was healed, and she was walking a mile a day now, something she could not do before that healing session.

Another one of the participants of my Star Energy Healing Group had a four-year-old daughter who happened to be a star child. Star children have come to the planet to raise the vibration higher for everyone. She was having difficulty at school and interacting with playmates. Her mother, who was a very gifted psychic, wanted a healing for her daughter and asked if I would be able to do this. I told her yes. My instructions were for her to bring her daughter, with her toys, to the home I'd rented in Tempe. We would sit on the sofa in the living room and talk while her daughter played with her toys.

Mother and daughter arrived, and we commenced our conversations. The daughter walked across the room and started to touch the sacred Navajo painting on the wall. At the same time, the mother and I both said, "No!" This startled the daughter, and she began to cry. The dear sweetheart melted into a temper tantrum from her frustration of not being given permission to touch the painting.

I walked into my office and came out with a one-inch polished heart-shaped rose quartz crystal. Handing it to the young girl, I said,

"Here, put this in your pocket. Anytime you don't feel good, rub it with your finger, and you'll feel much better." I also gave her a heart-shaped white paper doily to play with. The mother and I returned to our conversation. All of a sudden, there was an explosion of energy in the room that nearly knocked me off the sofa!

I looked at the mother and asked, "Did you just feel that?"

She replied, "Welcome to my world."

Quietly pointing at the daughter behind my raised hand, I whispered, "She's one of the new ones!"

That explosion of energy had been 100 percent pure love, and it was not contained in the living room or the house. It exploded out into the community. All these star children needed was love and to be happy. My hat was off to the mothers and fathers who care and raise these new children. For me, it was a deep honor to have channeled the healing energies for this star child.

Another interesting story about the sacred Navajo painting involves another healing client. One of the five bedrooms was a dedicated healing room, where I channeled healing sessions for clients. A young woman with left shoulder pain, headaches, weight gain, unable to do her yoga due to the pain, and intolerance to certain foods that caused stomach upset received a one-hour energy healing session. When she returned a month later for a follow-up session, I opened the front door, and her aura was glowing dazzling white. I thought I needed third-eye sunglasses just to talk with her. She reported her headache and shoulder pain were gone, she was back doing yoga, had begun to lose weight, and her digestive issues were completely gone.

On July 3, 2013, I received a trance channeling lesson via Skype with trance channel Summer Bacon[14]. I gave her a short demonstration of the mathematical star language. She was surprised, saying, "This language was coming straight from God Source. It's powerful. It bypasses the ego and goes straight into a person's subconscious." I hadn't realized how this light language worked in this manner, only that the language caused healing in a person. Summer gave me the protocol and exercises to deepen my channeling, and I began practicing every day.

---

14   https://www.summerbacon.com/

The progress of our spiritual journey is marked by an inner know-ing when it is time to participate and experience an energy modality that resonates with us. The 22-Strand DNA Activation was the next step on my spiritual path.

CHAPTER 4

DNA Activation

I HAD MET THE AWARD-WINNING MUSICIAN, Devara ThunderBeat[15], in December of 2012 at the Star Knowledge Conference held in Carefree, Arizona. Devara ThunderBeat is a Native American through her mother's lineage. The name "ThunderBeat" was given to her by Native American elders because of her ability to heal and awaken through the power of sound. She has traveled to numerous sacred sites around the world to redeem ancient knowledge and is a multi-award-winning international musician, composer, author, teacher, speaker, psychic, 22 DNA Activation Facilitator, certified Reiki Master, and pioneer in sound healing. And to top off this list of talents and abilities, she is an ambassador of the star planet, Sirius. I sampled her CDs in the vendor exhibit at the conference and purchased several of them. Her book, *Look Up: My Encounters with ETs and Angels*, is a collection of her stories of being transported onboard spacecraft her entire life since age four and is available for purchase through her website.

I felt the inner knowing that it was time to activate the 22 strands of DNA in my body and wanted it to be facilitated by Devara. On her website, she explained that the majority of the population has only two to three active DNA strands, and the other strands are dormant. When we come to a planet like Earth that has a lower frequency of dimension and the programming of human lifestyles, this blocks our DNA.

---

15   https://www.thunderbeat.com/

Therefore, we forget who we are, why we are here, and all our higher-dimensional capabilities. Most of the Crystal, Indigo, and Rainbow children have four to five DNA strands activated because Mother Earth has raised her frequency through our combined individual spiritual improvement efforts. These beings are now willing and able to come here.

Our bodies contain deoxyribonucleic acid. Commonly abbreviated as DNA, it is sacred, personal, and unique. It is the blueprint of who we are, where we come from, and why we are here on Earth. DNA determines our body type, behavior patterns, and potential diseases, and it holds our family genetic patterns and karma. It was passed down from our ancestors, and we then pass it on to those who come after us. In my case, I won't be passing my genetic patterns on because I don't have any biological children. I no longer have karma and strive to be conscious not to make more.

Devara says that the 22 strands of DNA are of etheric light-based DNA not visible under the microscope. This knowledge has been known for thousands of years. The ancient Egyptian priests and priestesses initiated 22 DNA activations in the temples. In ancient times, they did not call it DNA, but they identified it as the "22 golden light codes." In India, a Yogi receives many steps of initiations that activate their DNA, and it can take a lifetime. These Golden Light Codes were mentioned in the Keys of Enoch, in the 202nd section of the book. When a person was ready for the next step of ascension, they were attracted to the 22-Strand DNA Activation. In other words, you'll just know.

In Devara's Higher Density Blog of 11/23/14 article[16] referenced in the footnote below, she mentioned some of the benefits of a 22-Strand DNA Activation, including more energy and clarity, dysfunctional family and genetic karmic patterns clearing, immune system strengthening, a greater opening to connect with the Higher Self, and more.

Devara mentioned that this procedure activates dormant brain functions to their original divine function. One's frequency is elevated by bringing light into the physical body. People with DNA activations

16   https://higherdensity.wordpress.com/2014/12/28/devara-thunderbeat-the-next-step-activating-your-22-dna-strands-11-23-14-2/

begin to manifest the higher senses like intuition, telepathy, and clairvoyance. She explained to me that the session was about one and a half hours in duration. She records the session because information from a person's guides, ancestors, and angels come through, and the client verbalizes this during the activation. Only one activation was needed in a lifetime.

I didn't share with anyone where I was going and what I was about to do, and I contacted Devara, setting up the session for July 24, 2013. I drove up to Sedona, taking the Cottonwood route on State Route 260 from Wickenburg through Prescott. Her home was appropriately located near Thunder Mountain. Out in the middle of nowhere in the desert, I came upon a backup of traffic. I saw sheriff cars and a lot of officers carrying guns and rifles alongside the road and venturing out into the desert behind rocks. While I sat there, I heard loud thunder from above. For me, this was a good sign. The wait was about twenty minutes. When you're en route to an appointment, twenty minutes feels like twenty eternities. I called Devara on my cell phone to let her know about the delay and the confirmation of the thunder. She agreed it was a good sign.

I was met by her sweet Labrador retriever, Haley. As we entered her serene abode, Devara gave me a brief overview of the session. In the living room, with Devara standing behind and to the left of me, she began the ceremony. During the activation, we both saw colors and images and received information by clairaudience and claircognizance. Ra, the sun god, came through and bestowed his blessings. Much clearing was done from other lifetimes as a warrior dying from knife wounds, arrows, etc. She found a four-to-five-inch knife wound I'd sustained as a ninja. (Devara had not known I was a ninja in a prior life.) At one point, Haley barked and growled, and I followed by voicing the mathematical star language. Angelic tones came forth. I was in an altered state of consciousness. Suddenly, my body felt hot. Through my third eye, I saw a lifetime, like falling out of a boat and drowning. Archangel Gabrielle appeared and told Devara that I no longer needed to be a warrior. Instead, it was requested that I shine my golden light on the world. At the end of the clearing and repairing, I was taken to a beautiful mountain top of relaxation and peace. It was a very nice way to end the intense and effective procedure.

After the DNA healing and activation, Devara played her Chakra Healing CD while I lay on her living room sofa. It was peaceful and gentle. Afterward, she said, "Barbara, you should see your eyes! Go look in the bathroom mirror!"

She was right. My eyes sparkled with beauty. This was my physical evidence and confirmation of an amazing healing through DNA activation. Although it takes from three weeks to three years for full activation, I felt different already. We went out to dinner at the elegant Italian restaurant, Dahl and Di Luca, in Sedona. I enjoyed my favorite Italian dish, manicotti. Afterward, I drove Devara to her home and then headed back to Tempe.

I drove home very tired, really not knowing how I would make it back. I kept praying, asking my angels to keep me awake and safe. In retrospect, I should have stayed at a hotel in town. I arrived home around 10:00 p.m. and went straight to bed, then woke up tired the next day. Devara had said it would take a couple of weeks to recover. She'd recommended that I keep close to home and venture out only when needed, such as for grocery shopping. She was right. It did take two weeks to recover. In that time, I drank water. Lots of water. I asked people not to hug me at the Star Energy Healing Group events. I was being guided to keep this healthy boundary around me, knowing full well it would be over and I could return to hugging people the next month. I continued to present the Star Energy Healing Groups in Chandler for the rest of the summer and into the fall months while Barbara South provided the channeled angelic music.

The producer I'd met at the Braco event in the spring contacted me and arranged for me to give a Star Energy Healing group event in Sedona, Arizona. Unfortunately, the venue had a mold infestation and was shut down by the health department. I was given a list of venues in Sedona. The first one I called was the Sedona Creative Life Center. I felt the vibration of this place while talking with the room coordinator. Barbara South brought her Omnichord and speaker. I drove us up to Sedona. The producer made the hotel arrangements in advance for us.

The Sedona Creative Life Center was a beautiful place set in the red rocks of nature. Its architecture reminded me of Frank Lloyd Wright's style. The room for the group healing was perfect. We set up about fifty chairs for people to receive the energies.

Before we began the evening event, I noticed two women—a blonde and a brunette—arrive together to experience the healing energies. I spoke briefly to the blonde woman. She told me her friend never came to any events in the Sedona area. However, when the brunette woman saw the advertisement on a bulletin board in one of the village establishments, she looked at my photo and said, "I must see this woman." I took this story as a humble and pure compliment.

After a brief introduction, Barbara began channeling the angelic music. My Higher Self took over my body and moved my arms in various symbols. In an altered state of consciousness, I walked around the room and stood behind people as my Higher Self guided my hands to move around the participant's heads, touched their shoulders very gently, or made circular movements around their bodies. The mathematical star language was playing in my head. As I returned to the front of the room, the music stopped. I sat down and spoke the language. When the transmission was complete, I helped people return to their bodies through a visual image technique. I answered questions and shared channeled information.

When the event ended, the brunette woman came up to me and told me she experienced something profound. Some time ago, she was abducted and taken aboard a spaceship and tortured. She helped others process and recover from similar experiences. She felt she had already healed from her trauma. During the mathematical star language, all the memories came flooding into her consciousness. In her mind, she said, *Oh no!* All the memories then melted away. She found her true and complete peace. From that, she said to me, "Barbara, you're doing good work. Keep it up." I felt deep gratitude for her sharing her healing experience with me.

My next step in my spiritual journey involved my interest in making extraterrestrial contact. I have no fear of meeting extraterrestrials; however, I will have to put forth the effort to do this, especially if I want to meet the Arcturians.

CHAPTER 5

QHHT®:
Meeting the Arcturians

I N SEPTEMBER OF 2013, AFTER reading a couple of books[1718] about extraterrestrial beings known as the Arcturians, I was guided to contact them in person. This would be considered a CE-5—close encounter of the fifth kind—experience, according to Dr. Steven M. Greer[19], because it was human-initiated contact.

Steven M. Greer, MD is an American ufologist, retired trauma doctor, and is considered the father of the Global Disclosure Movement. Born in Charlotte, North Carolina, he became a medical doctor and specialized in Emergency Trauma Medicine. In the middle of his successful career as an ER doctor, he left medicine to devote the rest of his life to the disclosure of extraterrestrial contact and spacecraft technology. Dr. Greer founded the Center for the Study of Extraterrestrial Intelligence and authored several books and films on these subjects. What resonated for me was that Dr. Greer had initially trained to be a transcendental meditation instructor. He combined spiritual consciousness with ET contact, enabling humans to make peaceful and gentle communications with our star nations. In my opinion, this was the way to establish a mutually respectful and lasting relationship with extraterrestrial beings.

---

17   Milanovich, Dr. Norma J., Rice, Betty, and Ploski, Cynthia. *We the Arcturians: A True Experience*. Athena Publishing, 1990.

18   Miller, David K. *Connecting With the Arcturians*. Light Technology Publications, 2012.

19   https://siriusdisclosure.com/

From Wickenburg, I drove to the camping spot I'd gone to the year before. Telepathically, I was told by the Arcturians they would contact me during my sleep. Although I was hoping to see them while awake, I said, "Okay." I set up camp and ate a late lunch while reading David Wilcock's book, *The Synchronicity Key: The Hidden Intelligence Guiding the Universe and You*[20]. I felt a divine presence in the woods and spoke to the trees, expressing my gratitude. I thanked God for everything. Walking around the area, I found four heart-shaped rocks on the ground—three partially buried and the fourth one on top of the ground. I was told to take the one on top, their gift to me. They must have remembered I left them two moonstones and a rose quartz crystal last year on the large extraterrestrial head-shaped rock in this same area.

Just after I settled into my tent for the evening, it rained. No mosquito bites. No implants, as far as I could tell. I practiced my Kriya Yoga, then went to sleep. It felt so good to be lying this close to Mother Earth. I felt safe alone in the woods.

I woke up during the night and looked at the stars, seeing zillions of sparkling white diamonds on black velvet. We are very blessed to behold this beauty with our eyesight. I lay back down and returned to sleep until waking with my alarm for my thyroid supplement. I had no recollection of being on a ship or meeting a star brother or star sister. I was disappointed that I didn't make contact. I got dressed, ate breakfast, and broke camp, then drove back to the ranch.

In her book *Look Up!*, Devara ThunderBeat shared how she'd found out about her "missing time" extraterrestrial encounters through a session with QHHT® founder, Dolores Cannon, in January of 2004. I decided to talk with Devara about my experience in the woods, and she suggested I look up Dolores Cannon's website[21] and find a Quantum Healing Hypnosis Technique℠ (QHHT®) practitioner for a regression hypnosis session. I found a female Quantum Healing Hypnosis Technique℠ practitioner in Gilbert named Virginia. I wrote down her name and phone number to contact her when I returned to Tempe and left the

---

20   Wilcock, David. *The Synchronicity Key: The Hidden Intelligence Guiding the Universe and You*. Dutton, 2014.

21   https://www.qhhtofficial.com/

note on the kitchen counter as I walked into the living room to practice my Kriya Yoga.

During the last part of my yoga meditation, my third eye opened. I saw myself leaving my tent as a large, narrow pyramid-shaped space-ship landed in the clearing at my campsite. Two large, luminescent-looking Arcturians came out of the ship and walked down the ship's exit ramp to greet me. They were humanoid with human features for my comfort. I walked up and inside of the ship on my own accord. Then, I saw myself on a table surrounded by Arcturians looking over me as procedures were done. There was no pain or discomfort, even when a long, large metal probe was inserted into my left upper outer thigh. I asked the Arcturians what was done to me. They said they had upgraded my light codes and prepared me for the trance channeling of them on the BlogTalk radio program that evening. I felt love. Not once did I feel threatened or not welcome. It was as if this were a regular thing I did. Hmm. I left the ship and returned to my tent. At the end of my Kriya Yoga, the color blue was very deep and expansive in my mind's eye.

While speaking with Lance on the phone, I told him I did not have an experience with the ETs in the physical 3D realm but instead saw this movie in my third eye. I was disappointed from my expectations. He agreed I did indeed go on the ship and said more was going to come to the surface for me. That afternoon, I realized the scar on my mid left thigh was from an implant removed from me at age four. The area did not itch nor have discomfort. I remembered waking and sitting up, looking at the implant in my leg. The female being said for me to lay back down. They did not want me looking at this.

Implants are given to humans to assist the health of the human body. We are exposed to all sorts of chemicals and substances in our environment, food, and water that can adversely affect the functioning of our cellular processes. Who gives us these implants? The Higher Self does. That part of us that was merged with God/Creator Source, and at the same time, comprises a group of beings who are with us 24/7. They maintain the human form and energy systems necessary for us to occupy these vessels. A couple of days later, I returned to the house in Tempe and called the QHHT® practitioner named Virginia.

I did not do any research about Dolores Cannon and her QHHT® modality. Virginia told me the sessions were private and lasted about four to six hours, followed by a debriefing, and I would receive an audio recording of what was said during the hypnosis. We scheduled my session, and she sent me the preparation information by email.

Virginia drove to the house in Tempe, and we sat in the living room as I told her my life story. Afterward, I lay down on my Reiki table in the healing room, and Virginia began the induction. I felt comfortable and at ease. Virginia was a Level 1 practitioner. It was very easy for me to trust her and the technique because I had done the inner work to learn to trust myself. When we trust ourselves, we trust others using our discernment.

I was shown a past life where I saw myself at the foot of the cross where Jesus had just died. My name was Jeremiah, and I was taught by Jesus. The purpose of this past life was to love and support Jesus by talking with people, sharing how to love, how to forgive, and how to live a wholesome life. People came to me. As we progressed through this life, I saw scenes where I was a much older man. People looked up to me because I was compassionate and had an understanding that people who do bad things didn't understand why they were doing it. There was a reason for this bad behavior, to help the other person learn more about loving himself or herself. The ones I spoke with were thirsting for this information because Jesus was not among them anymore. This past life was a good life with family. I died peacefully with my loved ones around me.

Virginia called forth my Higher Self to speak with her, and my Higher Self said the purpose of showing me this lifetime of Jeremiah was to remind me of the teachings of Jesus and to help others in this current lifetime. The teachings of Jesus were important in my current mission.

A couple of days after this session, Virginia called me and said, "I've never met a Higher Self like yours. I'd like to meet them again. Would you be willing to have another QHHT® session?"

Since the first session was a very pleasant experience for me, of course I said, "Yes!" We agreed for me to come to her home office for the second session later that week.

People can experience and remember the time before their birth during meditation and energy healing sessions. Another way was through a Quantum Healing Hypnosis Technique[SM] session with a trained facilitator. This second session revealed the healing gift I'd brought with me into my current life.

We had just explored one of my parallel lives as a researcher and data collector of other planets, a life shared in detail in chapter fourteen, titled *Time Travels: Exploration of Lives Remembered*[22]. At this point of the session, I found myself in a new scene looking at a ball of light—an egg-shaped object that was milky white and translucent. Here is the transcript from that session.

Virginia: Are you small or large compared to this light?

Barbara: I'm part of it. I'm on the outside looking in. Like it's right before me.

V: Are you getting ready to step into this egg-shaped light?

B: Yeah, it's like I'm going to go inside. Like I'm going to come into it being born. Oh, this is how they do it!

V: Do you have a sense of yourself? Can you look down and see your feet?

B: I'm consciousness, getting ready to go into this form and become human!

V: Did you make the decision to do this, or did someone tell you to do this?

B: It's like a collective decision. I'm all prepared. I'm ready to go. Everything is all set.

V: Is there anything you are bringing with you?

B: All my gifts. All my skills.

---

22   Becker, Barbara. *Time Travels: Exploration of Lives Remembered*. Barbara Becker Books, 2018.

V: And what are those gifts and skills?

At this point, I began speaking the healing mathematical star language that I channeled as my Higher Self spoke during the monthly Star Energy Healing gatherings I facilitated for groups of people.

V: So you're bringing language with you?

B: Yes.

V: Are you being prepared to be Barbara?

B: Yes, very much so.

Virginia asked the Higher Self to come forward, then: She wants to know more about you. Who are you, and how can she bring more of you into her daily consciousness?

HS: We are a collection of love, frequency, of consciousness, of beings, entities, planets, stars, all the power that emanates from the Great Central Sun, all-knowing, all-loving, all-correcting, all-being. To incorporate us into Barbara's being is for Barbara to just be herself. We are here. We are not separate from Barbara. She is not separate from us. That is what she needs to know. As you know, in our incarnation as humans, we forget. Yes, and more and more of this is being peeled away.

V: Is there a name or visual image you could attach to yourself so Barbara can make requests and have conversations with you on a daily basis?

HS: The WhiteOne.

V: Can you help to reveal the specifics of her ET experiences?

HS: Yes, all she needs to do is go into meditation, request it, and we will provide. Visuals, sensations, information—all she needs, all she desires.

V: She feels she is a commander of a starship. What is her role as a star commander?

HS: To explore. Her ship is what you would see as pyramid-shaped; however, it's not vertical. It's horizontal. Very much this is an exploration ship with lots of other star beings on board, performing and gathering information, teaching, learning. Many schools are on this ship. She determines where to go next. Receives information from Command. All based in love. This is all based in love. Very, very much so.

V: Is there anything else she needs to know about being a star commander that will help her in this incarnation?

HS: She can draw strength upon this, that she knows exactly what she is doing.

V: I imagine there is a lot of leadership in that role.

HS: Yes. This is why people on Earth look to her for guidance as she sits there befuddled, "Why are they staring at me? Why are they looking to me?" Because she has this leadership, and they know it because they are on the ship too. This will be helpful for her to put closure to that questioning.

V: So, these people are recognizing Barbara subconsciously as their leader?

HS: Yes.

When a QHHT® client listens to the audio recording of the session, downloads of insight come through into the conscious mind. For instance, I realized, *This is how they do it!* Then, I came to understand that there was a group of beings guiding the process of consciousness embodying into a human. I further understood we have the ability to place our consciousness into an energy form (here on Earth as humans, as the egg-shaped light), and this was done with thought. "It's a collective decision," means I have met with my guides, council of elders, beings of light, angels, and so forth to draw up the game plan, so to speak, preparing me for my missions on Earth.

This part of the session answered my questions about trance channeling my Higher Self and the star language that was not indigenous on planet Earth. Also, the information affirmed for me that the language indeed was a gift. I wrote about the opening of the mathematical star language in my book, *Enclosure: A Spiritual Autobiography*. An audio sample of the language with healing can be heard on the Streaming-ForTheSoul.tv SuperPowers show interview with host Karl Fink on YouTube.[23]

While we are given our missions and contracts before we come to planet Earth, there are times when we discover our missions don't necessarily match up with our human-generated plans and intentions. My next experience illustrates this concept.

---

23   https://www.youtube.com/watch?v=FDnuqdNXs3A&t=1s

CHAPTER 6

Return to the Ranch

I 'M SHARING THE FOLLOWING STORY because it explains how we are not in charge of our lives. For the most part, it seems so, but there are times when we realize we are not. We may be called into the "office" for a conference...

I was contemplating offering a "Celebration of Life" blessing to anyone with a relative who was about to cross over. I had been told I have the ability to channel the energies where the soul can transition out of the human body with ease, comfort, and love. Having heard about terminally ill people being scared during the dying process, I called the various hospice facilities around the Valley and met resistance to my form of service. I subsequently found out that the hospice industry had gone "corporate," and if you're not working within the predefined treatment methods of the company, then the services are not wanted. This realization was depressing to me.

I talked with other healers who had tried to offer similar services and had been met with resistance too. It was presented to me that another angle might work. If I could learn a way to approach the hospice corporations on their terms, using language they are familiar with, then I might find an avenue to be of service. Even though I had hospice volunteer training, I really didn't want to become a hospice nurse because it required tuberculosis and coccidiomycosis testing, which is an old paradigm that I was no longer part of.

A dear friend of mine and energy worker, Janet, contacted her female friend who used to work at a hospice corporation and could revise my proposal letter for presentation to potential facilities. When the edits were completed, Janet came over to the house I rented in Tempe to discuss the proposal and her involvement in providing the same service too.

Sitting at the kitchen table, we began our discussion when suddenly I began to feel weird. I told her, "I don't feel well. It's like I'm between two dimensions."

Janet, who can see spirits and communicate with people who have crossed over, saw my guides standing behind me as tall, large, golden beings.

I told her I felt faint, and my energy was lowering.

She said, "Place your hands on mine."

Then I felt like I was going to pass out and fall down, so she helped me walk over to the living room sofa, where I lay down. Janet initially sat on the sofa next to my feet as I entered into an altered state of consciousness. With my eyes closed, I became aware that I was out of my body, hovering over myself and marveling that I wasn't breathing. I was in complete respiratory arrest.

Janet was guided to walk over to the side of the sofa, behind my head, and began toning. This went on for about five minutes, she concurred later.

Then, just as suddenly as I'd gone away, I returned to my body, sat up, and said, "Okay! Where do you want to go for lunch?"

The expression on her face was like a deer in headlights. I had no memory of what had transpired, just that I wasn't breathing for a period of time and now was back, energized and hungry. Janet had no clue either.

For several weeks after this event, I felt sad. I thought I had experienced a potential exit point. An exit point is where the soul is given the opportunity to leave the human body and not return. This can happen during serious illnesses and severe injuries. I knew I wasn't done with my missions on Earth, and although I would ask my guides for the meaning of what had happened that day, it would be two years before I learned the answer. For the time being, I dropped the idea of helping people in hospice.

As I offered my services as an energy worker and angel communicator, clients were steady but not enough in numbers to sustain a living. In September, I contacted my feng shui consultant, Lisa Montgomery. If anyone could read the money energy in the home, she could. When I told her about the lack of sufficient clients to support me, she said she would call me back after she checked my chart, as she was finishing up a consultation with a client in her store in Scottsdale. About twenty minutes later, I picked up the phone, and she yelled, "Get out of there now!" Through her mind's eye, she saw a huge red stop sign. "If you don't move now, you won't have the money to buy gas for your car!" She was dead serious.

I sat shaking my head in disbelief and confusion, not understanding why this would be happening. "Love what you do. The money will follow," they said. "Keep positive and in joy. Others will seek you out," they said. After all, I'd released old money programs, ancestor energies of lack, struggle, and pain. This should have been working, but it wasn't. This was not making sense to me at all.

We came up with a strategy to determine my next move. The only answer was to move back up to the ranch. In my mind, I was reviewing what had occurred so far: No money, no work at the ranch, moved to Phoenix area for work—guided to leave the well-paying job and go into self-employment. No money, no work in the Phoenix area, move back to the ranch. If this wasn't a recipe for insanity, what was? Logic tells us not to go into self-employment without a considerable amount of money saved and clients lined up for months. I knew I couldn't go back into the corporate world or nursing. Those doors were slammed shut for good. There was only one thing left to do. Trust God.

I put most of my furniture on Craigslist. All of the pieces sold within a couple of days, confirmation that it was time to move. I went through all my stuff and asked what to keep and what to let go of. I packed the house and called the movers. While on Skype with Peter, who was in Switzerland at the time, I told him I was moving back home to Wickenburg. I gave my thirty-day notice to my dear landlady and then moved back up to the ranch on October 31, 2013.

On November 22, 2013, I facilitated the Star Energy Healing Group to West Valley Center for Spiritual Living in Peoria, Arizona. It was a cold, rainy night. This was the first time I saw and felt a mischievous entity fly out of one person and across the room to another person. Although it tried to challenge me verbally, I did not let it sway the channeling of information, nor did I bring this experience to the group. I knew changes in the group gatherings needed to be done.

After settling back in at the ranch, I moved the Star Energy Healing group to a choir room in a Universal Unitarian Church in Surprise, AZ. This venue was about thirty miles from Wickenburg. The groups were small. Sadly, I had to let Barbara South go. It wasn't fair to her to not have large groups and be able to compensate her appropriately. I took her to dinner and explained the best I could. I truly appreciated her musical gift of channeling the angels. It was a good fit for my channeling of the healing energies. I felt I had to downsize and keep it simple—be a solo act.

I was guided to use a portable Bose SoundLink speaker with an iPod for music, and I contacted the renowned sound healing artist, Jonathon Goldman. He granted me permission to use his album, *Frequencies*, for my group sessions. We found his music to be conducive to bringing participants to a state of peace and tranquility for the mathematical star language transmissions. Jonathon's music was a good match for group healing.

My dear friend, sound healer, music therapist, former psychiatric registered nurse, Reiki Master, and drummer, Joan Pritchard, contacted me by phone from the Seattle, WA area to tell me she was told by her doctor that she needed a heart valve replacement. She wanted to know what I thought about it. She was finding it difficult to make a decision to undergo heart surgery that would give her about a year more to live or to not have any procedures and allow what will happen. I tuned in and shared with her that whatever decision she makes will be the right one. There was no wrong decision here. She told me those words brought her comfort. With that, she decided to go on a dream cruise to Alaska and return to have the heart surgery. Her doctor gave her the green light. Joan told me later she thoroughly enjoyed herself on that trip. I'm so glad she went and was able to enjoy the beauty of our Earth and her magnificent creatures.

Joan was the friend that I was about to visit at her home to trim her rose bushes in 2008 when Peter—the man who sat next to me in traffic school—asked me out to lunch. It was difficult for Joan to trim her bushes with her rheumatoid arthritis. This act of kindness was something I wanted to do for her. When my Higher Self told me to say yes to sharing a meal with Peter, I understood the rose bush trimming could wait one more day. It was a good decision.

In November, I received news that my massage therapist, Nani Tadina, had died at home. I was waiting to hear when the services would be, sad she was not in human form, but I knew she was okay. She'd been trying to contact me. My hummingbird glass ornament now has a broken wing where it sits on my windowsill outside my bedroom.

Three days later, I went to Nani's service and started to cough with phlegm draining from my sinuses to the back of my throat, while Anthony, Nani's boyfriend, spoke about her. I went to the ladies' room, then stood in the lobby asking my Higher Self if I should leave now or go back into the service. I walked over to the table that had a collection of Nani's collectible angel ornaments and statues. One of Nani's relatives who gave the eulogy asked if we would take one as a memento of Nani. I did not see anything that appealed to me. I looked to the back row of statues and noticed an angel statue lying on its side, behind a plant. I reached over to place it upright and noticed it was a porcelain guardian angel statue holding a star. I instantly knew Nani wanted me to have it.

On November 13, Peter and I held a yard sale. It went well, except for one lady who left her newborn in her car with the heat running on high. When she opened the back door and I leaned in to place the box of items she'd purchased from me, I saw a baby with sweat pouring down its forehead and covering its face. I asked the mother to take the baby out of the car to cool it off. She refused. I asked her again with more emphasis. The mother refused and said she would adjust the temperature. She turned off the heater. I became upset, then left my body very abruptly, and my Higher Self and the physicians took over. I channeled the language, and my arms were up in the air, making symbols.

People were watching me. I slowly came out of the trance. People were trying to ask me questions, and it was hard to talk. I wasn't fully conscious. I regained consciousness. In the meantime, the mother drove away. I felt I was prevented from noting her license plate to call the police. I knew I hadn't left the baby. There was a part of me that was still with the baby. WhiteOne said the baby was healed, and adjustments were made. I felt very frustrated that I didn't and couldn't do more. Later that day, I spoke with Lance, the shaman, and he confirmed the baby was healed and the mother received an adjustment in her brain so she will take better care of her baby.

I participated in Gma's intergalactic meditation teleseminar.

This was the "Corridor of Golden Light With the Galactic Council."

The opening scene from Gma was composed of multi-colored dolphins and whales, elders, archangels, mandala, suspended star systems, new planets, merged sense of being, gratitude, light, love, purified waters, and riding happy and laughing deep into Lemurian temples and golden pyramids.

I found myself enveloped by magenta and golden light. A wormhole portal opened, and I went feetfirst through a curved gold light path with the colors of magenta and blue-violet. I held a black rod about six inches in diameter and six feet in length. Then, I was in my whale form with Gma, diving deep before going up in the air. We worked on the Fukushima nuclear power plant, standing in the middle of the reactor in building four and three, feeling vibration all around. My mouth was wide open and smiling with joy, love, and gratitude. *I'm on vacation,* was my thought, beaming magenta and gold light around us.

Gma suggested that if you used a pendulum for answers, first ask if my name was Barbara Becker. If I got a no answer, I needed to sweep my auric fields head to feet, wait a couple of minutes, then ask again.

The next month, on December 8, at the Feast of the Holy Mother at Gma's intergalactic meditation teleseminar, Gma said the master numbers were eleven and twenty-two, as they have been in the month of November as well. Eleven shows the connection between all that was or will be, as brothers and sisters. Gifts are Protection, Right Use of

Will, and Harmony. The twenty-two was the Builder, the Square, and the Realization of the God-Self in All. Gifts: Rewards and Blessings were included in the theme. The focus of this teleseminar was Mother Mary, an archetype of the divine feminine birthing a cosmic thirteenth-dimensional being that brings to us a higher level of consciousness awareness regarding a new cosmic creation for the birth of the path of 2014.

I was holding a rose pyramid quartz and clear blue quartz crystals and saw three pyramids at the bottom of the ocean. There was energy and intense gold light. I could hear the mathematical language. I saw a whale spiraling, blessing all humanity and star beings. I was feeling all the trials, challenges, and suffering of all, and this was transmuted above the Earth, one with all. It felt like we were gone for hours. I had heat in my whole body. I did a transmission of the healing energy with the mathematical star language. Grandma said I gave an accurate description of what had occurred. The temples were about receiving an anointing for Earth and spiral consciousness awareness. She suggested I speak the mathematical star language while pouring water onto Mother Earth.

My friend, Joan, was in the intensive care unit, sedated and on a ventilator with a leg infection and heart failure. I contacted her telepathically, and she said she would "return as good as new."

In the summer of 2013, I came upon another master teacher through my metaphysical searches on the internet. Maureen J. St. Germain taught the 17-Breath MerKaBa meditation from the work of Drunvalo Melchizedek. Now that Maureen had published her 17-Breath MerKaBa Meditation course on DVD at the end of 2013, I was ready to activate my light body through this modality.

CHAPTER 7

My MerKaBa Activation

D ETERMINED TO REMOVE *ALL* BLOCKS to my prosperity once and for all, I started the MerKaBa Classic Flower of Life 17-Breath Meditation course with Maureen J. St. Germain on December 31, 2013.[24] I wanted to know what had happened to me that I could not or did not have the ability to see, hear, or know information for people.

In my mind, I heard, *"Just trust, Dear One, we will help you in this skill. Do not worry or feel you cannot receive the messages. And yes, in a lifetime as being a clairvoyant in a time where you and others were suppressed, great suffering was endured by you. You were burned in a bonfire in front of the whole community, and no one came to your aid or assistance, for they were fearful the same would happen to them. You must forgive them in order to heal this wound."*

On January 2, 2014, I activated my MerKaBa (light body) with Maureen guiding the group. I felt an intense pulsation on the top of my head that lasted for more than an hour. Two days later, I did the MerKaBa activation again. Maureen included her Higher Self Communication technique in her MerKaBa course. I asked my Higher Self yes or no questions about unimportant and insignificant actions to establish and foster a communication link between us. Soon after, without even trying, I experienced the neutral and the no response during a card game of solitaire. I knew a shift had occurred in me because I became

---

24   Now available on DVD at https://maureenstgermain.com/home/

claustrophobic at a restaurant when Peter and I sat down in the booth. After insisting that Peter sit across from me, I felt much better. I prayed for help from my angels. I needed people to purchase my services. I woke up every morning thanking God for everything, then doing my MerKaBa meditation every morning and Kriya Yoga meditation every other day, with qi gong, tai chi, and other meditations.

On January 14, Gma's galactic teleseminar with the Mother Mary and Lord Krishna energies began. I immediately felt Gma in my body as my head moved just like hers, back and forth. I could see golden light pouring down on me from above. I saw Mother Mary with golden light emanating from her heart and palms. My head rotated to the left and then to the right. Lord Krishna came, and I saw and felt more golden light. I held a large cobalt blue diamond cone and inserted it into the hole of a large cobalt blue star-shaped crystal. I saw more colors. I remember going to Einsiedeln, Switzerland, to the cathedral dedicated to Mother Mary in this meditation. Then, I went to Peru and unloaded a dump truck of gold coins onto the plaza in Lima. All the homeless children filled their pockets with the coins. It was delightful to see their eyes filled with such surprise.

I saw many tubes of light energy in brilliant colors. Gma came into my body, and I was in hers, filled with unconditional love. I cried tears. I then asked Gma to show me herself as a dolphin, and she did. I was in a boat, and she came up and smiled, then kissed me on my forehead. I said, "Thank you."

Mother Mary came again and handed me a red rose. My head dropped back as I looked up to the ceiling and saw brilliant magenta light pouring down on me. I then was high above the pyramids and saw a white light at the apex. I began speaking the mathematical star language. My head dropped down, and through my third eye, I saw a pink light beaming from my heart.

Gma said we were all given a new heart connected to the star, Sirius B, where a manifestation portal was located. We could now manifest anything we wanted. It was 2014, and we were expanding and shifting quickly that year. Now, we could sustain our rays of energy in our everyday walk along our path. The blue silver ray was constant. Athena said we went through a blue diamond and out to the galaxies.

We visited Gma's white star planet and hung out with her. The Orion being of light attended us, and we went there. The Galactic Federation of Light gave permission to the Arcturians to produce the rainbow ray, clearing and negating the effects of the chemtrails, so anytime we saw a rainbow and there was no rain, sending our loving energy to the rainbow gave it more fuel.

I'd awoken two nights in a row with heart palpitations, and Gma was with me the last night it happened. Cat recommended magnesium and potassium—make a green smoothie 50 percent fruit and 50 percent green veggies.

On February 8, 2014, my dear friend, Joan Pritchard, died in Tacoma, Washington, with her family at her side. Several days later, just before sunrise, I walked out to the promontory point in the desert behind the ranch, where one can catch an unobstructed 360-degree view of the horizon. From this high hill, one can look down on the Sombrero ranch houses. Just before I began a drumming ceremony in Joan's honor, my drum made a sound. I knew it was Joan saying hello to me. I missed being able to talk on the phone with her, catching up with each other's activities and insights. It was such a joy to hear the laughter and enthusiasm for life in her voice. I can still see her joyful smile in my mind.

On February 9, 2014, the wonderful energy worker and clairvoyant who had witnessed my "conference with my guides" in Tempe came up to the ranch for a healing, and I received one from her through energy work and a Thai massage. I cried during the massage as emotions surfaced. I had a sudden realization that I must leave the Sombrero ranch without Peter. Where was this coming from?

A client from the previous year came for a healing on February 11. I spoke about his tics and the underlying metaphysical reason for them. They could have been because he was afraid to be seen. He was very relaxed after the doctors on the other side worked on his brain and his thought processes. I did not see any tics during the 1.5-hour session, just the occasional normal right arm movement when one sleeps. He snored during the session, so I knew he went very deep.

February 16 was the first day after my forty-five-day training period with my Higher Self, WhiteOne. I now could ask serious questions and receive answers very clearly and quickly. I asked if it was time to move and was told no, but that the information would come through at the right time. Everything was being prepared and would come into my reality soon. My Higher Self suggested I continue packing. It had been over a year since I'd last spoken with any member of my family. I thought fondly of them and wished them well, knowing we would all be together again. I just didn't know the circumstances and when.

In meditation, I was shown my wealth garden and its flowers, animals, and more money trees, forming a beautiful orchard. I received confirmation of my steady spiritual progress and continued to practice every day to hear my Higher Self answer questions and give me guidance.

CHAPTER 8

Higher Self Communication

ON MARCH 13, 2014, MY friend Joyce arrived at the ranch. Peter, Joyce, and I ate dinner together. Later, Joyce and I talked after we got our pajamas on. As we lounged on the two queen-sized beds in the third bedroom, she was wondering what was next in store for her life. We stayed up late, and I did a tarot card reading for her in her room. I also noted intuitively that she was carrying entities with her and that they were not the nice kind. These entities came from a guy(s) in prison and had attached themselves to her energy fields. Joyce's ex-husband worked in a prison in Arizona. I asked her if I could do something to help her release some stuff around her, and she immediately said, "Yes!" She sat up on the side of the bed, and I channeled the language as my hands moved around her head and upper part of her body, then down the lower part, and then I held her ankles momentarily. I stood up, and just above her head in three areas, I clapped my hands loudly, startling Joyce.

Afterward, she felt much better and lighter. She said, "Maybe this was the reason I was supposed to come up here, for a healing and removal of this stuff."

I agreed with confirming tingles in my body.

The next morning, I woke up at 5:30 a.m., showered, and ate breakfast with Peter. Joyce had said she would get up around 8:00 a.m. and later told me at breakfast that she'd heard a gentle voice say, "Time to wake up." When she'd looked at the clock, she had ten more minutes.

Five minutes later, she heard the female voice again, "It's time to get up now." I confirmed with Joyce that the voice was of Barbara, the woman whose family built this home seventy-seven years ago, and she was sleeping in her room.

Joyce and I walked out to the pool house and talked for another thirty minutes. When we walked back into the house through the kitchen, a black helicopter flew by the ranch in plain view from the large picture window in the breakfast area. Peter stood with us in the kitchen, witnessing this event too. Joyce turned toward me and asked, "Men in Black?" I motioned for her to follow me and took her to the bedroom to explain about the black helicopters. (Recently, Peter and I had noticed an increased number of medical helicopter flights over the ranch.) Now, if my MerKaBa program that was running made me un-noticeable to the black helicopter ETs, then this must mean Joyce and I together were triggering the surveillance. When I walked out to the garage, I heard one of the ETs tell me telepathically, *"You understand us, Barbara."* The voice was not threatening nor had any sinister vibration. My Higher Self, WhiteOne, confirmed these were benevolent star beings watching over us. I hugged Joyce goodbye with teary eyes and watched her drive off, down the Sombrero Ranch road to State Route 93 on her way to Utah.

March 17, my father's birthday, was the first time I did not call him to wish him a happy birthday and tell him that I loved him. I did, though, send him my message in the ethers. I whispered it outside, letting the wind carry my blessings and best wishes. I knew he was preparing to leave this dimension and physical realm to return to what he was before he came and agreed to be my father. I heard him reply, "I love you too."

On my birthday, I facilitated the Star Energy Healing Group event, clearing and blessing the room before I entered. There was so much energy that I could hardly breathe until I adjusted the energy level. Five people came, but I later saw that it was a message telling me to change the group to teleconferencing. During the channeling where I completed the individual healing, I felt Archangel Michael enter my body. I knelt down on one knee, prayer hands and bowing to everyone, and felt his large wings widespread. The love emanating from my/

his heart was immense. I was guided to get up and sit in the chair, then channeled the mathematical language as WhiteOne spoke. Then Archangel Michael spoke to the group through my vocal cords. When I came out of the trance, I did not remember Archangel Michael speaking until one of the participants mentioned it.

On the drive back to the ranch, WhiteOne said to me that they would come through and speak in the English language for the groups and answer questions. The following day, I asked the WhiteOne if we needed to practice the channeling. They said no.

On April 1, 2014, Peter expressed his desire to practice qi gong with me. I was surprised because it had been a while since he'd joined me. It was windy and cool outdoors, but we had a wonderful qi gong. Every time we do qi gong together, we feel awesome afterward. He noticed he was able to breathe much deeper and easier too.

On April 5, during the night, I felt my bed shaking during an earthquake while in the between state of asleep and awake. I checked on my computer for Wickenburg, and there had been no earthquakes reported.

On April 21, 2014, at about eight in the evening, I was lying in bed preparing to go to sleep. I heard a voice that I recognized as Don, my childhood friend, Dianne's, husband. He had died from a battle with cancer and had a distinct Texas accent. I never thought about Don, so this "other side" communication from him was unusual. The times I'd visited Don and Dianne in Houston, I truly felt honored to be in his presence. He was genuine, happy, and a very compassionate person. He loved cats too. I could feel his presence and acknowledged him, then asked, "What is it?" He asked me to call Dianne and let her know he was fine. I told him I would call her in the morning, and if she didn't answer the phone, I would leave a message, asking her to call me. If we did talk, I would see how the conversation went to determine if she was willing and ready to receive a message from her late husband. If not, I wouldn't say anything. I didn't push this type of information on anyone. It's considered proper spiritual etiquette to wait for permission or receive an invitation to share. After this conversation with Don, I looked up his obituary on my iPhone internet application. There, I found his memorial service was April 21, 2013, exactly one year ago!

The next morning, I called Dianne and left a message. The last time I'd spoken with her was in the summer of 2013. She never called me back, and I let it go. There was more to this event. I would not truly appreciate the magnitude of Don's message for two more years.

Five months later, I did a little research and found that on September 1, 2014, Dianne wrote a note on a funeral home online obituary memorial book for Don. I knew Dianne would have called me back. We had always called each other back eventually. We had been good friends for many years. It felt sad to not have those times again. For me, this was one part of life that sucked. People come into our lives for a reason or a season.

On April 26, 2014, Gma's intergalactic teleseminar focus was on the evolution of the self on all levels. Gifts are sovereignty over the Self, Elevation, and Right Use of Power. Gma said we would be traversing time and space into new levels of ascension for ourselves, all of planet Earth, and beyond. This was to prepare for ascension takeoff to new planetary systems and galaxies. We were celebrating with the whales and dolphins and integrating the full blossoming of all that had been planted previously. The transport vehicle we used was the Flower of Life, inside the cosmic egg of creation of All That Is. The Flower of Life can be found in all major religions of the world and contains the patterns of creation as they emerged from the Great Void. Gma went on to say that everything was made from the Creator's thought. After the creation of the Flower of Life and the Seed of Life, the same vortex's motion was continued, creating the next structure known as the Egg of Life. Gma went on to say this structure forms the basis for music. It was also identical to the cellular structure of the third embryonic division creating the human body and all of the energy systems, including the MerKaBa (Light Body).

Gma asked us to visualize the color magenta, which was the color of the Cosmic Christ on the thirteenth dimension with the cosmic whales. We also visualized the color violet for the highest spirituality and gold for self-mastery. Jesus and St. Germaine assisted us in our meditation. She said Jesus was now working under his galactic name, Sananda, which was the name adopted after his resurrection.

Gma said Joseph, the father of Jesus, was believed to be St. Germaine of the Violet Flame. His mother, Mary, upon her Assumption, became an archangel and was now the twin flame of Archangel Raphael. I entered the ascension meditation with Gma by myself while I listened to the recording on April 3. I went out and came back briefly because someone coughed on the recording, but then I saw Grandma Chandra as a golden dolphin. After the recording, I asked Gma what had happened. She said in my head, *"I assisted in changing the tones of the Universe to one of love, joy, and bliss to raise everyone's vibration on Earth and other planetary homes for all beings. Athena said we went to the Arcturus' ashram and were also in the Great Pyramids in Egypt."*

On May 10, 2014, I asked my angels for help in manifesting the money to live on my own and take my business and services to the next level. My Higher Self said everything I was doing was working. Everything would line up with synchronicity. I asked, "Do I move now?" WhiteOne said, "Not yet." WhiteOne told me I wouldn't be at the ranch by the end of summer. I did not have the town or city name where I would be moving to in Southwest Colorado. On June 13, 2014, I was told by the WhiteOne that I'd negotiated more time to be in Arizona before I moved. I had a new time frame.

On August 12, 2014, the skies were gray as Peter departed for the airport at 9:50 a.m. to fly to Switzerland and visit family and friends. The limousine was a little late. After the car was out of sight, I sat down in the living room and cried. The memory of leaving Hoyt and what he'd felt after I left him came into my consciousness. This is the program of abandonment that we humans must resolve. After the feeling washed away from me, I decided I must move forward. I couldn't go back.

While lying in bed one warm July night, Gma's frameless photo on my nightstand fell onto the shelf below. I knew instantly that she was calling me and asking for my attention. Of course, I said yes, knowing it was time for work. Off I went to sleep. The next day, I received an email confirmation from Cat that Gma had indeed moved her picture on my nightstand. Every night, I asked Gma to take me with her on our missions and could hear her in my mind. The work we did was not to be in my conscious mind. All I needed to know was that it was for the highest and greatest good of humanity and beyond.

One day in September, I was driving home from the grocery store in Wickenburg when my Expedition's serpentine belt broke on Tegner Road at the intersection of Bralliar Road. Suddenly, there was no power steering. Turning the wheel felt like turning a ton of bricks without a forklift. I felt the surge of fear overcome my body like a rolling river of water filling a desert wash. I prayed hard and asked God, Archangel Michael, Archangel Metatron, and Ascended Master Morea to help me get my 2000 Ford Expedition up the serpentine road on the hill and into the garage. The amount of energy surrounding my body grew immense. Up the hill we went and into the garage. I sat for a moment and embraced the fear, then let it wash away. We made it! I focused on transferring the groceries into the house and being grateful for everything that had been given to me.

Later, I went out to the pool and swam. I remembered the tough spots I had been in before and realized everything would work out. Then I had a good cry, feeling the aloneness in this physical reality. I missed Peter. When I released this, I stepped out of the pool, sat down in the pool house, and focused on everything I was grateful for. I reconnected to my Higher Self, the light, and the love. Faith and trust reenergized my beingness.

There was a theme there—serpentine belt, serpentine hill. Rattlesnake hill was where the ranch was located. The snake was about change. I was changing. My life was changing.

I watched a video of Dr. Greer and his technique to make contact with extraterrestrial intelligence. The video showed a group of people sitting in chairs with Dr. Greer as he began the meditation with a small Tibetan singing bowl his wife had gifted him. Through my third eye vision, a green saucer-shaped spaceship came toward me and stopped right in front of me, in the living room. During the meditation, I felt someone physically stroking my left arm. I asked and received confirmation that a star being was in the living room with me, making physical contact very gently and lovingly. I was at peace and grateful for this interaction with an Arcturian traveler.

Gma's galactic teleseminar, on June 20, 2014, was about opening the Summer Solstice of prosperity and the ascension gateway. We were celebrating the fruition of all that had been planted these past few months and initiating a worldwide house clearing of lack from our consciousness. This opened the way for the Unity Consciousness of Prosperity teleseminar, where we activated the Crystalline Grid of our group mind consciousness by opening the Portal of the Great Light that connects and receives Light from the higher dimensions, connecting our auric fields to the activation of prosperity for everyone.

We took this journey with the dolphins and the whales from Sirius B, diving into the depths of the waters to refresh and refortify for this higher expansion and opening of the Prosperity Gateway. Our guides on this journey were Sanat Kumara and Legions of the Great Central Sun. Lord Sanat Kumara was an "Advanced Being" or Ascended Master, regarded as the "Lord" or "Regent" of Earth and humanity. He was thought to be the head of the Spiritual Hierarchy of Earth who dwelt in Shamballa. The legions of the Great Central Sun are a source and center of the all-pervading, mighty *I Am* presence. It was a point of integration of Spirit and matter, a central concentration of God consciousness and the release of light, life, and love to all creation.

The master number for this meditation was twenty-two—the builder, the square, the realization of the God-Self in *all*. The gifts we received were blessings and love. The vehicle for this journey was the six-pointed star inside a circle. The six-pointed star was two interlaced triangles, a symbol that was variously known as the hexagram, or the Star of David. It represents the transmutation of the lower three chakras of matter into the higher three chakras of intellect and spirituality. The colors of the first three chakras are red, orange, and yellow. The colors of the upper three chakras are blue, indigo, and violet. Red was the complementary color of blue, orange of indigo, and yellow of violet. We focused on visualizing violet and green.

In this teleseminar, I saw the star of David in light form and went through it. Then I went into my whale form in Hawaii, then found myself in Alaska among the icebergs. I traveled into the Great Central Sun. The left side of my body tingled, and then I was in Colorado. There were beings around me, and I definitely felt I was in Shambala.

Gma confirmed everything, saying I'd placed a star-point portal in Colorado. I was going around the planet opening star gates with her, which was allowing more prosperity in. Gma said I was one of her favorites to work with because I'm fun.

On September 18, I woke up and discovered the house had no water. In fact, the whole ranch had no water. I asked my angels to intervene and help me solve the problem. The next day, I called Wickenburg Pump & Supply. The owner, Walt, came right over and began diagnostics. It took him almost two hours to determine it was the well. He sent his crew over, and they brought the well pipes up two hundred feet with a crane. The impeller had deteriorated and broken apart. A new one was installed. At two in the afternoon, the water was restored at full pressure.

I performed an angel reading via email and sent it to the client, then celebrated the water by jumping in the pool and hugging it. Much gratitude! A shower after swimming felt so good. We appreciate more what has been taken away and returned.

Over the internet, on September 28, 2014, we celebrated our sixth anniversary of meeting each other. Peter told me the same thing every year: "And still going strong!"

On October 13, 2014, a door opened. Virginia, the QHHT® practitioner who had facilitated my first two sessions, called and shared with me her vision to open a medical clinic with doctors and alternative medicine practitioners, such as QHHT®. She had already picked out an office in Durango to rent and said her QHHT® practice was picking up. People were driving three hours for sessions. She and another QHHT® practitioner swapped sessions for each other with the same questions to see if the same answers were given. When she'd asked who she could go into business with for this alternative work and medical office, her Higher Self had said, "Barbara Becker." She told me that my healing work would be a good match for QHHT®, as it would give the client tangible evidence of the healing. She offered to pay for my QHHT® training and the parapsychologist license exam, and I would pay her back and move to Durango. She agreed with me that I would need to meditate on this. I decided I would ask WhiteOne in a QHHT® self-session facilitated by me. I told Virginia I would put myself under hypnosis and speak with my Higher Self that afternoon. Synchronicity showed up, as I had already planned to hypnotize myself to get guidance on where to take my healing career next. Some people call this coincidence.

I lay down on my bed and relaxed into the deep trance level of hypnosis. Then I was taken off the planet, up into outer space, and swooshed down rapidly into the ancient town of Pompeii, Italy. This experience felt much like doing a "find location" in Google Earth. I saw myself and Virginia as two men working together, laying the metal pipes for the city's water supply. In 1995, I had toured Pompeii and Ercolano, Italy. Now, I understood why I had instantly recognized the exposed pipes under the cobblestones of the street, pointed out by our private tour guide. In my past life, Virginia, as a man, had fabricated the pipes.

In the trance state regression, I served as negotiator and architect for the system. I also saw that Virginia and I, in that life, had been very successful in business together. At this point, I asked my Higher Self if QHHT® was in alignment with my soul path and agreements. They replied, "Yes, very much so."

It was during my Kriya Yoga meditation on October 17 when I saw a lotus flower opening in my third eye. I saw bright flashes of light and felt the sensations in my body. I felt very relaxed after I came out of my meditation. Walking outdoors felt peaceful. I was beginning to feel that I was at another crossroads in my life. You know, that feeling that something was about to change.

CHAPTER 9

*Quantum Healing Hypnosis Technique*SM: *Becoming a QHHT Practitioner*

W HILE ENJOYING AN OCTOBER AFTERNOON coffee in the sunroom of the ranch house, I spoke with Peter about Virginia's proposal of me facilitating QHHT® sessions in Colorado. I shared that this was an opportunity for me to expand my healing work and that he and I could live in several places, such as Switzerland, Colorado, and Arizona. He shared with me that he was making arrangements in Switzerland for us but wasn't specific. We agreed to continue our relationship even though we wouldn't be living together the entire year. I loved him very much. He was not the same as me and brought so much into our relationship, a diversity that was causing growth for both of us. He shared with me that his green card expires in 2017, only two years away. We would start up the weekend open houses next month to sell the ranch. Holding me in his arms, he said to me, "You need to do what you love, and that's your healing work." I told him I appreciated his support. I did not realize how prophetic his message would be for me.

Virginia and I would have some hurdles. WhiteOne said people would come to help us. I had to take the QHHT® course—twelve online lessons in two weeks—and take the exam. I would need to study and take the Colorado parapsychologist license exam also. And I would need a place to live, snow boots, and a winter coat if I moved before or during the winter.

Elina Sharp, who owned the Open Door 1 & Too shops, invited me to give angel readings for the public during the Front Porch Festival in downtown Glendale, Arizona, on October 18, 2014. Peter drove us and graciously helped me set up and take down the booth. I had a wonderful time giving angel readings to the public. I was exhausted by the end of the day. Little did I know that while I was giving angel readings to the public, Dolores Cannon, creator of the Quantum Healing Hypnosis Technique℠, passed over from her Earthly existence.

I soon discovered that Peter had purchased a one-bedroom apartment in Aeschi, our favorite place in Switzerland, and had been keeping it a secret to surprise me; however, the things he was telling me were not adding up. He said he was going to rent an apartment next summer. I told him I knew he'd bought an apartment. He laughed. I could see the stress of keeping it a secret leave his body. I told him that I appreciated him finding a place for us in the most beautiful place in the world. We both loved Aeschi bei Spiez when we were there in 2009 and 2010, and we saw this as a summer place for us to live. It was a custom apartment, and he'd ordered everything last April. We had fun looking at all the information and photos about the apartment that was being built over the months to come. He was tickled that he could not hide the truth from me.

I was staying present in the moment, working on learning QHHT®, planning on finding a place to live in Colorado, and being in business with Virginia. I didn't know how this would all come about, but I trusted my angels, guides, and WhiteOne would figure it all out.

On October 27, 2014, I began the QHHT® certification course. I was told by WhiteOne that I would take the exam at the end and pass with flying colors on the 3rd of November. It took me a week to complete the course, and I did pass with a high score. A couple of days later, I signed up for the original support forum developed by Candace Craw-Goldman with Dolores's blessing. I was learning more as I read the case experiences shared by other practitioners. This was gold!

On November 9, Dolores's memorial service was held in Arkansas. In my bedroom on the ranch, I recited a mantra that a practitioner had shared on the private forum. I began my Kriya Yoga and went into a deep meditation. Suddenly, Dolores came to me in the form of a ball of violet light in the middle of my bedroom! I felt so much love that my tears flowed. She said I would do really good work, and she was glad I had taken the course. She said she would be with me when I facilitated the client sessions and gently guide me. I could not contain the amount of powerful love she blasted upon me. It was truly something so profound.

Part of the training to become a QHHT® practitioner was to offer about thirty sessions for free. The practitioner needed to become familiar with the nuances of hypnosis and guiding their client in Dolores's technique. I decided thirty-three people would help me become acquainted with this hypnosis work.

On the morning of November 14, I heard my angels say to me, "Come outside, Barbara, right now." I had been asking to see a spacecraft that was not from this Earth, one that was not a back-engineered military rendition. As I walked out to the pool and looked up, I saw a perfect angel cloud. At that exact moment, a military jet flew over, heading higher in the sky, due northeast. Shortly afterward, a realization overcame me. This was a spacecraft piloted by a star being, and it had been made to look like a military plane. I surmised that if our military people could make and pilot spacecraft, then why couldn't our star brothers/sisters mimic our old-fashioned technology too? WhiteOne confirmed my realization, and chills swept throughout my body.

The day after Thanksgiving, I was at a crossroads again. Peter was mad at me for not bringing more money into our household. He'd been carrying most of the load and developing increased symptoms of stress and anxiety. He was right. I'd done all my marketing, gave free sessions, published a weekly newsletter, and engaged in social media, and was ever so grateful for Ann Albers's referrals for angel readings. Now, I was at the end of the road. I had to be patient and take action at the same time. I prayed for God's help. Ann Albers came to my mind. I knew God wanted us to take action, and we would be provided for, so I placed my full trust and faith in God.

I asked Ann to help me get the word out, and in early December, she published my ad for free QHHT® sessions. Six people contacted me that same day. Within two weeks, I had my calendar full for thirty-three clients, and more people were contacting me. Soon I was booked up until May of next year! Thank you, God! Thank you, Ann!

I began facilitating QHHT® sessions in the middle of December. I could hear Dolores's voice just outside of my right ear and could feel her in the room. She gently guided me in her matter-of-fact voice, saying, "Move her to another day." This first client was a challenge for me because she kept analyzing with this expectation that she needed to see a past life. That wasn't what her Higher Self had in mind. She was shown a plethora of images that she would make sense of later when she listened to her session recording. She was a highly resistant person to this technique. I left wondering why the session was not as "textbook" as I had hoped. Maybe it was to show me that even I was not to have expectations of the client's experience under hypnosis.

On March 27, 2015, during Gma's intergalactic teleseminar, I saw gold light and golden temples. The floors, ceiling, and walls were made of gold. I saw the pyramids in Egypt and myself flying a spacecraft. I saw myself looking inside a glass structure building. Gma said I was looking at the portal that was being constructed over the ranch. It was 60 percent complete.

On May 3, 2015, in this intergalactic teleseminar, I saw Gma as a woman. She stood with a dress covered in eagle feathers. The feathers hung down from her long sleeves as she chanted and sang. I saw a very large white tipi and was invited to go in. I saw Chief Golden Light Eagle and Gma. I knelt down, bent over as Chief Golden Light Eagle held his hands on my head, and Gma held her hands on my back, behind my heart. The chief prayed and chanted, then I sat up, and he showed me a snake eating its tail. I then saw myself ascending inside of a spiral of golden light with blue light pouring down on me. This meditation was further initiation for me. More was opening in terms of my gifts and abilities to assist others in their ascension.

May 31, 2015, I asked Dolores to regress me for this bladder irritation-anger issue I had. I wanted to know the root cause. She was in her stuffed chair, and I was on my bed. Using the QHHT® protocol, I heard Dolores recite the script in an abbreviated format. I saw many images and asked WhiteOne to show me the root cause. I saw myself standing on the flagstone courtyard patio, urinating on it. Answer: The anger was from having to stay there at the ranch for another two years. I would continue to drink extra water as the WhiteOne guided me. I came up and out and thanked Dolores for her assistance. I loved her very much. She said she was proud of me, and I was doing good work with the QHHT® modality. "You're coming along very nicely," she said.

By June 16, I felt stuck at the ranch, not moving forward in service to others. I had to wait patiently, as God provides in the perfect moment. I asked my Higher Self to guide the people to me for assistance in the ways I could provide. I knew I was taken care of, and the funds would be there. I was going to the QHHT® second-level course and believed it, even though I had no evidence showing me it would happen. And then suddenly, everything came together.

On July 11, 2013, Virginia picked me up at a gas station off Interstate 17, at the Carefree Highway, and drove us to Springdale, Arkansas, for the QHHT® second-level, three-day course. We drove to Amarillo, Texas, and stayed at a Marriott hotel, where Virginia used her award program points for the room and breakfast. We also attended the QHHT® Practitioner Reunion the day after the course. Then we left Arkansas and headed to Amarillo to stay at the same hotel. The following day, Virginia drove me to the Albuquerque, New Mexico airport for me to complete the last leg of the trip home while she drove home to Durango, Colorado.

In Amarillo, that first night, Virginia had facilitated my third QHHT® session. Although a person only needs one QHHT® session for the remainder of their life, for some people, it is a challenge to relax down into the deep level hypnosis, as Dolores and I have both found. For those people, having another session convinced the ego that this modality was safe and informative. Additional sessions afforded the ability to do further exploration of same or different concepts and experiences. A session benefits the ego because its job is easier when the client knows his/her direction, life purpose, and answers to pressing questions. It was in this session that Virginia and I learned more about me. We decided not to go into a past life and instead focused exclusively on speaking with my Higher Self to get answers to important questions. My Higher Self was accessed immediately in deep-level trance hypnosis from the code word I had given Virginia two and half years earlier. Here is that conversation:

Virginia: Barbara had an unusual experience in the home she was renting at the time. An energy worker named Carol, who visited with her, saw Barbara's guides standing behind Barbara as she shared that she felt a strange sensation of being weak and disoriented. She would like to know what happened.

Higher Self: Well, dear Carol saw *us* standing behind Barbara. We were calling her back for the moment. We needed to see her in council because there was some indication that she did not want to continue her mission. So, it was very important that we have a little chat, so to speak.

V: What was the indication that Barb gave? Was that in the physical realm or in the spirit realm that the indication was given?

HS: It was in the spiritual realm. Barbara was not consciously aware of this, of course, because she did not understand what was transpiring in her body. We gently guided her to a higher realm and had to make adjustments in her body, which she did see that she was in what we call a partial suspension. And this was done because we had to make adjustments in her, and we had a very constructive and productive talk.

V: Can you share with Barb, in this realm, what was her hesitancy for not continuing her mission?

HS: She did not really want to go back to the ranch, and we had to remind her that there was important construction, if you will, that had to continue there, and we needed her there. And that was why we were the ones who changed all the finances and the situation that she was in, in Tempe. She had finished construction of the portals—the gateways, if you will—in the Tempe area of the Valley. That was done. She'd agreed to do that, and now we asked her to please go to a special area in the desert, an area where it is conducive for transportation of souls to go to different points, wherever they are needed, different places of the solar system—the galaxies, if you will—other planets and star systems.

V: This new construction project at the ranch, she was hesitant to go and do that. Can you tell me more about this construction project at the ranch?

HS: She's very much an instrument, if you will, the unconditional love that is required to construct this portal. It's all constructed with unconditional love. She is doing this with others. There's a great number of others participating in this. It's a group effort, if you will, and we will say that it is about 90 percent complete! We think she will be pleased with that number. It's going to be a little bit more for her and then she will be moving to Durango, Colorado!

V: Will there be construction projects in Durango, or will she be focused on different types of work?

HS: Oh yes, in addition to her sessions in the Durango area, there are more portals to be constructed there. She's going to be changing energies up there. She will be working with others, of course. And this is all part of the assistance for the earth.

V: The construction of the portals is done with unconditional love. Why does her physical body need to be there? Why can't they be built from a distance? We know energies can travel great distances. Love can travel great distances. Can you help us to understand the mechanism of why the physical body needs to be there?

HS: Yes, yes, my dear. Well, she holds a frequency. And the human body holds a frequency, and that is the requirement. She holds that. It's part of the matrix of the construction of the mechanics and the energetics—the mechanisms that allow entrance and exit. Of course, this is not in the physical realm.

This is through dimensions; intergalactic travels. It's a very beautiful place.

V: You mentioned more than just Barb is involved in the construction proj—

HS: There are thousands!

V: How many of these portals are on the planet?

HS: Goodness gracious! Let us see here… Two thousand to three thousand. We can't make an exact number there because they are in different stages of development. Sometimes, there's interference.

V: You mentioned after the construction project and going to Colorado? What is the timeline for her?

HS: Still not yet. We know she's wanting. There is part of her that says, "Okay, I will go along, and I know this will come about in the perfect timing." She has come to terms with that. And we are very appreciative of her being there in Arizona. She has more work there to do. She will be given the information. It will come, and it will be very obvious to her that it is now time.

Another interesting event occurred that I wanted to know more about on February 12, 2015, between four and four thirty in the morning. I was awoken from a deep sleep by loud sounds as if a spacecraft had crashed onto the tile roof above my bedroom. Then something boomed, like tiles crashing on the flagstone walkway outside of my bedroom. My heart raced. Since I did not hear anything else, I told myself I would look at the damage later in the morning when I woke up. Later, when I looked outside, I found nothing out of place or disturbed in any way. The answers to what had happened that day came during the thirty-fifth QHHT® session I facilitated. A psychically gifted oriental medicine practitioner's subconscious revealed this:

HS: There was sacred geometry being put over your house,

and what you were hearing was the shutting of this shape from one dimension to the other. Your house is being worked on as well, so you can continue your work at this house. It is being surrounded by sacred geometry. It needs work before you are to leave it. The physical house and land need work. It needs sacred geometry around it so you can leave it and move forward.

Barbara: Is this being done when I'm asleep?

HS: Yes.

B: Will this be done by May?

HS: Yes. You can't do all the work yourself. This geometry, we are resetting the house so that you can leave it. But the slamming was the geometry opening the portal and then shutting.

More sounds occurred during my sleep on many occasions that spring. One time, I heard a loud bang through the dimensions that sounded like a slamming closure of the lid of a steel trashcan. I listened further. Not hearing anything else, I soon fell back to sleep.

On July 17, 2015, in the Amarillo hotel, when I facilitated Virginia's session, I asked more questions of her Higher Self about the ranch portal.

Barbara: In my recent session, my HS mentioned the portals around the earth and that there are two thousand to three thousand, depending on the stage of construction and interference. What is that interference? How does that come about?

HS: There are many beings from many places that have come to this place in the galaxy to help with the growth. The portals are a necessary part, and this takes a lot of effort. It's not magical. It takes time and commitment and ability and resources to bring these beings in. Many cannot stay in Earth's atmosphere for very long. As helpers are shuttled in and out, contributions to the amount of work that is completed can ebb and flow. This is the source of the unpredictability of the building of these portals. There are many beings who have sacrificed their lives for this work because they have stayed in Earth's atmosphere and dimension too long.

B: Virginia's HS told me the ranch portal is very close to completion, more than 75 percent.

HS: You have been away. This is an example of unpredictability. It's very close to completion—more than three-fourths completed.

B: I wonder why there is a difference between two Higher Self's perception of the completion percentage of this particular portal?

HS: The chef knows the ingredients and how much time it takes to prepare, mix, and bake a cake, so they have one perception. Someone who is just watching the chef has a different perception because they don't know all the steps, the components, and the procedures to make the cake.

B: What is the most important time for me to be at the ranch for the construction?

HS: The work goes on when you are in meditation, when you are in thoughtful, open heart space, in addition to sleeping. When you are walking with a loving, open heart with the flowers, birds, and trees around you, this is helping to build it.

July 28, 2015, Peter left for Switzerland to visit his family while I stayed in Arizona to take care of the ranch.

On August 9, 2015, I listened to Dr. Greer's Glendale, CA 2015 CE-5 Intensive YouTube video twice that day and experienced a meeting with the Alpha Centurions. First, I saw a fuzzy alien face with large, elliptical eyes. Then I saw outlines of many humanoid people.

I now understood they were introducing themselves to me so I could become familiar with their features. They came with me to the ranch, and we spoke briefly. They asked me, "How can we be of service?" I replied very humbly, "How can *I* be of service to *you*? I give you my love and welcome you with peace. I ask for help in the only thing that's heavy on my mind, helping me to pay my car insurance premium tomorrow. I know this may be silly, but I'm in the third dimension and need to pay this bill tomorrow."

The very next day, I received the money in the form of a channeled healing client scheduling a session through my website. My gratitude soared!

I had another portal 3D experience on August 11, 2015. I went into meditation using the CE-5 initiative meditation with Dr. Greer and woke up an hour later to a loud crash on or in the house. The house shook! This home was made of concrete with twelve-inch-thick walls. The shock wave occurred at the moment I was coming out of sleep. It had felt like I just went into meditation, but it was an hour later.

A few days later, at 11:15 a.m., the power went out on the ranch— no water, no electricity, no air conditioning, and no gas. Then all of the electronics in the house went bonkers. There were noises, lights flashing on and off, and ceiling fans grinding. I ran around turning everything off, unplugging all the plugs, and lights turned on even though I had turned them off. I thought the oven was going to catch fire with the noises and flashing displays I was seeing. I looked outdoors and saw an arcing on the electric pole that looked like a small flame shooting out. I called the electrician, the fire department, and the electric company.

I had difficulty reaching Peter in Switzerland because the landline and my cell phone would not work. The firemen came after the electrician and stayed until the part burned itself out on the pole. I could not have removed the breaker switch next to the smart meter because it was jammed. I used ice packs on my head to keep cool during the hottest recorded day of the summer. The firemen told me to call them if I needed anything.

There was a storm the day before in the town of Aguila, twenty-five miles west of Wickenburg on Route 60. About twenty electric poles were knocked down by the high-velocity winds, so most of the electric company workers were there repairing the poles and wires. The worker who came up to the ranch told me he would try his best to find a coworker in Phoenix. The coworker had a cherry-picker truck to get the switch high on the pole back to its correct position and power the ranch. I was grateful for his kindness and effort.

The remainder of the day, I sat or laid with an ice pack wrapped in a towel on the top of my head and kept up with my water intake. It was so hot in the house. Remembering my first day in tai chi, I found strength in enduring the uncomfortable heat. About eight thirty that night, while lying on the living room sofa in my nightgown, ice pack on my head, the room lit up. I sat up and looked around, seeing bright lights coming toward the front of the house from the driveway. It was the electric company truck with a cherry-picker bucket on it! My hero had arrived!

It was a ten-minute job, and the kind electric company worker also realigned the jammed breaker switch for me on the electrical box. With the air conditioning now working, I was able to sleep in a cool environment.

I was finding confirmation and peace while reading Dolores Cannon's *The Custodians*, and my consciousness was expanding. On page eighty-one, Dolores came to me and said, "Your life is going to change now, Barbara."

During a MerKaBa 5D meditation on December 16, 2015, I saw a light tube coming down through my chakras into Mother Earth. Four Hathors[25] stood around me, front and back and at each side. My head was off my body as they turned my head to the right, facing my right shoulder, then to my left in 90-degree angle movements. My head was replaced, connected to my spinal column. My left nasal area experienced discomfort as an implant was installed. "Dear One, this is an upgrade for you and your light codes. We do not intend for your discomfort. You did request this. Insertion complete." Discomfort gone.

Each MerKaBa 5D experience was different. How can one describe

---

25   Hathor was the Egyptian deity most favorably disposed to help alleviate one's suffering, to provide comfort, and restore balance. https://www.ancient.eu/article/58/the-five-gifts-of-hathor-gratitude-in-ancient-egyp/

what cannot be described? The formula was simple: experience, trust, experience, trust. Rinse and repeat.

On January 10, 2016, Gma Chandra's teleseminar gathering involved the master numbers 11:11. The eleven shows the connection between all that was and will be as brothers and sisters. The gifts of protection and right use of will and harmony are bestowed upon us. Gma said we were in the fourth New Earth cycle, counting from the end of the Mayan calendar of 2012. This was the new age. We had accelerated our unity consciousness. We were *all one*. We had to choose to bring in the peace, joy, good health, prosperity, and love on all levels to the third dimension. Everything was reflected in and back into the whole. We were now more in alignment with our self and our life purpose. We used violet and white colors in our meditation. St. Germaine assisted us. Our vehicle for this meditation was the restored DNA strand. Grandma recommended her oils for assistance in the meditations. We used the dodecahedron for the embodiment of the etheric presence, which created the cosmic blueprint in continuous cycles downward from the Star World and into the heart of Mother Earth and then back up.

During this meditation, Gma was seen as a whale. I was on top of Gma, riding her whale form. We went into Mother Earth and visited military installations around the world. I then saw golden bands of light around Earth, causing everyone's vibration to increase and an increase in abundance for all lightworkers, translating to more clients coming for healing and guidance. People were awakening and wanting to work on themselves.

A gas explosion down the hill on Saturday, February 6, 2016, rocked Peter and me out of our sleep at 6:02 a.m. The neighbor who owned the land next to the Sombrero Ranch had broken the gas line during the construction of patio homes and the new neighborhood's infrastructure. The gas line fed the Sombrero Ranch because it was once part of the original six hundred forty acres in 1937. When the leaking gas reached the garage in the first patio home, the freezer had switched on and ignited the gas-filled garage, causing a huge explosion. When the explosion shook our ranch house, we both sat bolt upright in bed and then flew through the house. I told Peter to go outside and check the guest house to make sure the tenant was okay. Meanwhile, I turned on the television in the living room to see if there was a disaster of some sort being covered on the news station. Nothing was being reported. We donned our jeans and jackets and jumped in Peter's vehicle. Driving down the hill, we saw flames over the treetops. The fire had destroyed two cars and most of the structure. Thankfully, the homeowners were in Canada at the time. This story never reached the newspapers.

We had no gas to supply the stove and heater for our home for four days, so we improvised until the gas company brought up large bottles of propane gas on a long trailer. We burned mesquite wood in the fireplace to heat the house. They were able to connect bottles of gas to the main gas line feeding the ranch. I was impressed with the care and thoughtful attention for our comfort demonstrated by the Southwest Gas employees.

After two months of being bottle-fed gas, Peter negotiated with Southwest Gas to install a two-inch gas pipe from Tegner Road, through the town of Wickenburg, and down Bralliar Road, so if a future developer needed a commercial-sized gas feed, it was already established. Right-of-way permits were graciously granted by other businesses on Bralliar Road, including the community hospital. All ended well for us and future dwellers in the area. We came to realize that the tragedy was actually a gift for us and other people.

Later in the month, I was guided to enroll in Dr. Greer's webinar of Advanced Ambassador training, remote viewing with consciousness, contact meditation, CE5 protocol, and free energy device presentation. I did the meditation during the live stream and saw two star beings. I did the meditation at the end of the live stream and saw a rotating spacecraft underside. I felt I was being prepared to become acquainted with third-dimensional contact (CE5). I missed the first lecture, so I was waiting for it to become available to watch while learning about ceremonies of prayer, called *pujas*.

On February 29, Peter and I went to lunch at Paradise Bakery. While waiting for our salads, the music over the restaurant's audio system played a song that sounded like the Fibonacci sequence. I instantly recognized it, and it brought me an inner sense of joy while listening to it. Of the years we'd been eating at that restaurant, I'd never heard music like this. I had heard others speak of phenomena like this occurring when you make contact with extraterrestrial beings. Dr. Greer said that we could be contacted at any time.

I missed the first presentation of the webinar. While listening on February 29, I played the CSETI tones and the meditation with Dr. Greer. I did the thought sequencing. Before I started, my whole body became hot. I had to take off my track jacket. Then when I cooled off, I put it back on unzipped. At the end of the meditation, I turned on the magnetometer, and it registered red all the way to the end of the scale for about forty-five seconds. Then it went back down to the thirty-to-forty range. I walked around the room, and there was no spike in the needle. I thanked them for coming, even if I couldn't perceive them. I told them I loved them. My entire body had piloerection, otherwise known as goose bumps. I told them it's okay to come and visit me at night, and even to wake me up because I'd like to convey my love and respect, and of course, only if it's safe for them and they feel comfortable.

On May 1, I did another shamanic meditation. From the pool house, standing on the hilltop and looking out to the horizon of big puffy white clouds, blue skies, and green rolling hills, I walked barefoot down the sandy path that curved to the right slightly. I saw the forest surrounding the gentle stream that flowed through the area. I saw the cave across the grassy clearing. When I reached the bottom of the path, I turned my head up. To the right, I saw Angel Treasure on his painted horse. He was holding a spear with a dangling feather. As his horse walked down the path, coming closer, I saw the paint on his face. He showed me there was a situation that called for the warrior spirit within me. I bowed and hugged him. He handed me the quartz crystal. As he spread the blanket on the grass, I took off my clothes and walked toward the stream. There, I entered the water and lay down on the quartz crystal in the stream. Allowing the water to flow fast from my crown to my toes cleared and cleansed my soul. The toxins bubbled to the surface, and it was done. I rose from the water and walked toward the clearing, dried myself off with a white towel, and stepped back into my clothes. I placed the quartz crystal in my leather pouch hanging from my leather string belt.

Angel Treasure said, "You must go in there alone. I can't go with you. I will meet you on the beach."

I understood.

Walking into the cave, I felt the cold, wet stones on the bottom of my bare feet. Using the walls as my guide because there was no light source, I made my way inward. I could barely make out a shade of darkness that was lighter than the present one around me as I kept walking along the curved path. I saw a treasure box filled with golden coins and jewels but kept walking. I came to a cathedral formation of the cave, and inside a large vortex of energy and pure air showed a large hole in the cave. You could walk around the hole on a two-foot path, but that was not what one does when on a shamanic journey. I could feel that I was about to do something that would require courage and my trust. This wasn't like jumping into the Grand Canyon as I had done before while holding onto Angel Treasure's neck. Instead, another shaman appeared. He was of small stature, wearing feathers and a leather loincloth and holding a spear. I imagined if I didn't do as he said, I would feel the business end of that spear prodding my butt to move forward. Much like my life, moving forward was the theme.

"You must jump into the hole. You may die. You may live. It's your choice. Either way, you must jump. It's best to jump far and not hit the sides."

It was no good to argue with this man. I knew he was me. There was no hesitation on my part. I walked backward about fifteen feet and ran as fast as I could, tucking my feet and legs in as I left the ground and hurled myself as far as I could. The trajectory changed as gravity sucked me into the hole. I began spinning as I traveled through the vortex that became a wormhole, a portal to where I was to be. I lost consciousness and woke up later without memory, disappointed that I couldn't remember. I also knew something had occurred for my good. Some meditation journeys are just like that.

I left for Arkansas on June 5 to attend the QHHT® third-level course. My fellow student called me and said there were storms in the Houston area and that flights were canceled or delayed. I rebooked my flight through Denver, and this worked well. From Fayetteville, my fellow student and I took the recommended limousine service to Eureka Springs. I could feel the energies of the crystals underground. I really enjoyed practicing my tai chi and qi gong in the woods of the Ozark Mountain area. I cannot talk or write about the course because I signed a nondisclosure agreement.

I booked a room by myself because I didn't want anyone else's snoring to disturb my sleep. During the second night, I felt the crystal energies. While still awake, I floated above my bed and relaxed into it. Then I felt myself travel through my bed mattress, through the floor, and deeper underground, into the crystal matrix. This was when I drifted off to sleep, feeling immersed with the crystals.

The next morning, I woke up and had an epiphany. Emotional attachments, otherwise known as entities, were a hot subject with QHHT® practitioners because Dolores didn't believe they existed. I suddenly realized that even entities that are seen and experienced are still part of my reality; therefore, they are within me, not external or outside of me. That there was always something to learn from the situation. I finally really got it! This was why the Higher Self could and would take care of entity issues. My Higher Self can and will remove emotional attachments, and it's in alignment with the client's Higher Self because there is no separation. It's all love.

I then went further and asked my Higher Self, "Where is QHHT® going?" People are saying it's evolving into something else, where other modalities are needed in the QHHT® session. I knew instantly that QHHT® was going where it had always been…in Source! It didn't have to go anywhere, nor did extra modalities or techniques need to be added. It was already complete because it adapts to the situation, to the client, to everything! There was much going on behind the scenes during a session where other modalities were at play but not overtly seen.

The third level course in QHHT® was where Dolores, when she was alive, would check the practitioner's facilitation of a session. What was interesting was when I facilitated sessions, Dolores came through and said that I was doing good work and to keep facilitating these sessions as I was doing them. Not once has she said for me to go back and relearn the technique. This was especially true when she talked to me through a level-three QHHT® practitioner while I facilitated the session.

I love QHHT®, and I love my clients. Dolores has told me that I don't give up on my clients. Every one of my clients can go into deep hypnosis because they prove it when we do the fun exercise prior to their session. I'm going to be writing a QHHT® session stories book soon. I know I will receive guidance through circumstances and desire. The when is yet to be determined.

Life could be so darn frustrating at times. I continued to work on patience. It was June, and I was struggling with the financial piece of my life journey. If only there could be a class or modality that would help me finish this financial challenge within me.

CHAPTER 10

Blow to the Heart

O N JUNE 28, 2016, I participated in the free, online one-hour Soulprint Healing for Affluence class with energy worker, Carol Tuttle. Afterward, I walked into the dining room and noticed the energy flowing away from me in the form of arrows, then abruptly did a U-turn and found the arrows were directed toward me! I didn't realize my prosperity flow was outward bound. I'd been giving my money energy away and didn't even know it. This must have been at a subconscious level, maybe a cellular memory or in my DNA lineage. The hidden ancestral programs, patterns, and beliefs were up and running at full speed, creating an inward flow of struggle, pain, lack, and an outward flow of prosperity, elusively flying away fast and far from me. I know this abundant prosperity project still needed working on, so I signed up for the course. My Higher Self agreed to this purchase.

July 1, 2016, I began the course, and Dolores Cannon let me know she was glad I was engaging in this healing because this was one of my personal pieces that I'd chosen to work on in this lifetime. After the emotional freedom tapping (EFT) exercise for depression, I found a smile on my face. Wow! This was powerful.

Well into week two of Carol's prosperity and affluence course, I was shifting. My energy was shifting. I was releasing. I had the lowest energy day yet, where I couldn't do anything but manage to engage in my swimming program in the pool and home maintenance of painting the windowsills to freshen them for the new homeowner who would arrive and buy the ranch someday. The next day, I felt much better. I felt very happy and prosperous. Having the feeling of what you want is important in manifesting positive realities.

By week three of the Soulprint Healing course, my body ached all over. I was processing and drinking lots of water. Programs were being deleted, and old neuro pathways were being cleared out. Ride it out and drink water. The next day, I was feeling awful. The ache in my neck and back muscles was wearing me down. I did the Soulprint healing exercises and meditations to release old programs. It was hot, and I was tired. I looked forward to the fall with cooler weather. A couple of days later, I was feeling better as I headed to Phoenix to facilitate a QHHT® session. It was an amazing session. A little bit of a challenge, but the Higher Self managed to get through to answer questions and give messages and guidance for my client.

The roller-coaster ride continued. The following day, I felt yucky again, still clearing ancestral patterns, beliefs, and conditioning of lack, pain, and struggle. WhiteOne said I was doing good work. Swimming in the pool every day was healing for me. I love water, and it was so refreshing from this summer heat and my inner work. In week four of Carol Tuttle's program, I was feeling strong and steady.

On July 22, 2016, I woke up feeling good. Energy was higher. Peter was depressed. He was very worried but wouldn't tell me why. Something was up, but I couldn't put my finger on it. I did my best to maintain my steady, positive frame of mind. My mental and emotional perspective was much brighter, lighter. WhiteOne said my energy had shifted and continued to shift. Two days before he left, Peter and I made love for the last time before his trip to Switzerland. I was still not generating enough money to pay for a ticket, so I stayed home.

On July 26, I drove Peter to the airport and stayed with him for almost an hour. We ate lunch together. We kissed goodbye several times, and I told him I'd placed light around the planes, and special angels would be flying with him to keep him and everyone safe. He always had tears when he turned and walked toward the security checkpoint at Sky Harbor Airport. This time was no different. I watched him walk away down the hall, toward the gate area, until he disappeared. Then I turned and walked through the airport to the garage where my Expedition was parked. I drove back to the ranch feeling a part of me had gone with him.

There was a big storm on July 30. No significant damage. Electric was still working. Thank you, God. The pool was messy. I cleaned the filter basket and backwashed the pool. When I returned to reverse the backwash plunger, I discovered a rattlesnake under the pump tubes, about five inches from my right hand as I flipped the switch off. I jumped up and back. My fight or flight mode reflex kicked in. I went inside and Skyped with Peter. He recommended I throw some rocks near the snake and see if it would crawl away. I tried it, but the snake kept on sleeping. The pool water was draining fast, already about eight inches below the tile. Now my concern was about the pool pump damage and whether I was able to walk around the snake and pull up the plunger to reverse the outflow of water without getting bitten. I got the garden hose out and began filling the pool to buy some time. I took one of the snake poles we kept outside and lifted the sleeping snake, placing it gently behind the gas heater, then asked the snake to leave. It settled in and returned to sleep. I left the gate open and asked God to make the snake leave. I returned later, and the snake was gone. The pool filled up, and life returned to normal, or so I thought.

On August 5, I managed to get through a wall of tears and sorrow. I made chocolate cookies and felt absolutely wonderful afterward. The serotonin was flowing. I was feeling better and anchored it into my root chakra. Swimming was fun, and I meditated, still working on changing the old programs. I made slow progress, though I was able to daydream, and it felt good. My Higher Self continued to say I was doing good work.

The next day, I saw an Aladdin's lamp image in the clouds and made a wish to break through this money energy problem. I had to look at the money energy with my ex-husband, Hoyt. Money had been a major issue in our relationship. More correctly, it was the difference in our approach to money. At lunch, I said to myself, *Just let the memory be and appreciate the sorrow*. Maybe that was one way to look at it. I was determined to change my perspective. But how? On the one hand, I could say this was meant to be. I was meant to leave him. It was in the contract, that I knew. I looked at the high emotions around money with Hoyt. In 2004, I got a job and was able to go to Peru in December and then moved out of the house in October of 2005. When we divorced in 2006, he gave me a considerable amount of money as part of the divorce settlement. I remember when we transferred the money into my bank account, I'd felt strange. It felt like too much money for me. Now I understood it was too much for my energy to handle. I wasn't ready. This was similar to when people win the lottery. That amount of money coming in that fast is too much for a person's energy field. If the person is not disciplined and doesn't have a support system and plan in place, they usually end up with nothing.

In one of our meditations, Carol had us imagine a locked door in front of us. In our hand, we held a golden key that unlocked that door. We didn't know what we would see on the other side as we opened the door, and she asked us to be brave and unlock it anyway. At first, I imagined a treasure chest overflowing with gold coins that represented my wealth. I put that image aside and returned to a state of no expectations. I unlocked the door, opened it, and stepped through the threshold. To my surprise, I saw a large audience of my family and ancestors clapping their hands, congratulating me.

I asked, "What did I do?" They said, "You cleared all of the lack, pain, and struggle programs running in our DNA lineage since time immemorial." I replied, "Okay." Then I stopped, thought, and said, "Wait a minute, why me?" They replied, "We knew you could do it."

I returned to the group and completed the class for the week, then walked out to the pool area and sat in the pool house. I laid back into the chair, staring at the ceiling. In my body, I felt a release of the pressure around my heart. My body felt drained of energy and then it gradually filled back up. My energy increased. I felt lighter. Dr. Peebles channeled through and said, "God bless you indeed, dear Barbara! You have done the unfathomable again! We are so proud of you, my dear." I thanked Dr. Peebles and everyone, including my ex-husband, Hoyt, and sent him my love. I was now at peace.

Dolores Cannon contacted one of my QHHT® clients from the other side. She wanted Robyn to explore the Mandela Effect[26]. Recently, this phenomenon had sparked an interest in Robyn. She contacted me by phone. We both agreed that a QHHT® session could be done for exploration. An added bonus was for us to ask Dolores to come forward and give us her perspective.

We met at a hotel for the session, and I brought my computer and webcam on a tripod. We decided which questions I would ask. I helped Robyn to relax through the QHHT® script, and she allowed her Higher Self, which happened to be a high council, to come through. They answered our questions, and Dolores came forward, also a member of this council.

About a week later, I met Robyn at her house, and we created a video series with our commentary. Robyn then placed each video she edited on her YouTube channel. I thought she did a very good job of editing and creating a lovely series of experiential and informational videos.

On August 13, 2016, I returned home after grocery shopping and went into the kitchen to prepare a late lunch. I heard a loud noise out front and walked toward the sunroom, noticing the quail and white wing doves were screaming as they ran away. There was an old woman in a silver Toyota car, gunning the engine (pedal to the floor) for over a minute, parked in front of the house. I raised the window shade and watched her exit her car and walk up the stairs. She picked up rocks and placed them on the front porch, then walked around the house. She didn't ring the doorbell or even see me standing there in the glass window. She appeared to have no intention of ringing the doorbell or seeing if anyone was home. I was standing in the sunroom and staring at her as she walked around the house, toward the second master bedroom. I called the Wickenburg police. I asked them to come because there was a lady trespassing and acting bizarre.

Two police cars arrived (one being Joe, the former realtor Peter had introduced me to) within five minutes. I gave them a description of her, and they walked around to the master bedroom as she came around to the front of the house on the north side, carrying a large

26   The Mandela Effect is an unusual phenomenon where a large group of people remember something differently than how it occurred.

boulder. I was standing on the front lawn, near the entryway steps, and called the dispatcher, asking him to tell the officers she was now at the front of the house. She looked in my direction but did not approach or say anything. She sat down under the sumac, facing north. One officer drew his gun and held it behind his back as he approached her from behind. When asked what she was doing there, she replied, "I thought this would be a nice place to live because it's for sale."

I reminded the officer that the ranch *was* for sale, but by appointment only, and she was not acting normal. I gave Joe a large plastic cup filled with ice water for her, and they called the paramedics to examine her. The ambulance came and took her to the hospital for a psychiatric evaluation. The police officer stammered while trying to explain the situation. I told him I was a former emergency room nurse, and this made it easier for the officer to talk. I was told she was on psychotropic medications, so I said a prayer for her and hoped she received the care she needed. I felt sorry for her. She seemed so lost.

Speaking with Lance on September 1, 2016, I shared with him the episode with the woman who came picking up and relocating rocks on the property. His interpretation was from a shaman's perspective, of which I received confirmation as he spoke:

"She was you. She was representing the ancestral lineage of struggle, lack, and pain programs that was probably over one thousand years running. She was picking up the boulders representing the old stories, beliefs, and programs that you're releasing. The boulders represent blockages, heavy thoughts, and beliefs that have weighed you down. She was removing the boulders from the fence gates as a symbol that you are releasing it all. There's no more division, as noted by the fence. She was bringing this up to the doorstep of your mind. The police represent 'monitor or police your thoughts.' You gave yourself compassion through the glass of ice water. Also, it represents that you are getting rid of the old ancestral stuff through the emotional release that you are doing in your energy work. She, in her psychotic state, represents the mental instability in your family that has gone on for generations because someone, a long time ago, did something, and it 'drove the child nuts.' By going to the hospital with the paramedics, it represents that you are clearing out and healing yourself and your family. Gunning the engine represents that you are clearing through your body, and it's effective. Coupled with the snake encounter, it all makes sense that the energy work you're doing is indeed working. Beautiful confirmation of a significant shift occurring. Congratulations, Barbara!"

Lance went on to say, "The woman's response to the police officer about why she had come up to the ranch was, 'It just seems like a nice place to live.' She's talking about your mind."

I posted the photo and story of the rattlesnake on social media, and Zeysan sent me a message on August 21, 2016, that read, "I think snake form was what you need. It would be a lifelong practice. My friend taught me much of this. She was a wonderful lady. If you choose, find her performance of snake. Get a DVD and take it real slow where it can be done that way, and do it as exact as you can, but remember, it will not look like hers. Feel all in order to achieve the move. Snake form was one move. I don't know if you remember, but Cansu was learning this."

On September 13, I worked on my QHHT® book by preparing the chapters, organizing paperwork, and then did my tai chi, qi gong, and Kriya Yoga. I made pumpkin butter cake that came out perfect. Peter met with Swiss investors in a four-hour meeting to purchase the Sombrero Ranch. The money part was cleared for the Swiss investors, and they were looking to come to Arizona on the 1st of November. It appeared we would be moving to Switzerland sooner than I'd thought.

On September 14, my mother called and left a message, saying it had been six years since she'd heard from me. It was really only three and a half years. My mom wanted to know what she had done to deserve me not communicating with her. She said she could see I had a website, I did healing work, and she wondered why I didn't talk with her. How could I call myself a healer? She cried and hung up. I knew I was being tested. I felt her pain, and I cried. I couldn't go back, at least not yet. If she only knew how hard it was for me to stay away.

On the last day of summer, September 21, 2016, I sent Karl Fink a birthday wish, and he responded with an offer to interview me on the Superpowers show for my QHHT® service! I was delighted. The interview was done one week later and uploaded to YouTube from his video platform called Streamingforthesoul.tv[27]. I'm very grateful for Karl's project and the creation of videos for people to learn about near-death experiences, superpowers, healing messages, and stories.

It was the 23rd of September when I woke up with a dream where I was holding a cat and had a white dog with me. We walked over to a small pond. The dog motioned to me that he wanted to go over to the water, and I went with him. He jumped into the water, struggled to swim, then allowed himself to drown. He was on the bottom of the lake, and I was very upset. He was there for some time, and I managed to put the cat down and told it to stay. I went in, picked up my dog, and brought him to the surface, where he became alive and turned into a spotted white dragon the size of the dog. This was when I woke up.

This dream represented the part of me that was loyal to my spiritual journey. The water represented my spirituality. By not resisting and allowing myself to surrender my ego for it to be integrated with the Higher Self, this meant the death of my ego. Although we don't kill our ego, it's more about integration. The cat represented the quality of my independence as an awakened being. The dog returning to life was symbolic that we never die. The dragon with the spots was telling me that I have more inner work to do. Eventually, the dragon will become pure white as I develop my higher consciousness.

September 27 was our eight-year anniversary (Switzerland was ahead nine hours), and this was the email I received from Peter:

> Good morning my dear
>
> Happy Anniversary. 8 years, it was as it was last year.
>
> I hope you can enjoy this day.
>
> I have to do something today. The water was turned off because the town was putting a new pipe into the road and today house number 10 and 12 will be connected.
>
> Talk [with] you later.
>
> I love you,
>
> Peter

---

27   https://streamingforthesoul.com/

We talked later that morning via Skype. I missed him very much. Little did I know this would be the last time I spoke, saw, or felt the Peter I'd come to know and love.

By the 1st of October, I had not heard from Peter by email or Skype. Six days later, I sent an email asking if he was having trouble with the internet because I hadn't heard from him. He wrote back, saying simply, "I'm traveling." There was no mention of love nor his name. No words of comfort were written to allay my concerns.

It was the 8th of October, and I'd had eight days of intense left trapezius muscle spasms and pain in my upper back. It dragged me down to the point that I didn't want to do anything. I'd been applying heat and resting. I had finished the Soulprint for Affluence course with Carol Tuttle and was receiving more requests for QHHT® and channeled healing sessions since the interview with Karl.

On October 12, I experienced a five-minute period of feeling like I was between the dimensions—that faint feeling. My guides said I was called into a meeting. I returned, and then I felt fine. I asked the WhiteOne, "Where is Peter? What is going on?" They said that Peter was with them. Now I understood that we were in conference on the other side for what was about to happen.

I woke the next morning feeling good and made my coffee and breakfast, hoping one more time that I'd hear from Peter. There'd been no response for days. I sent an email telling him that I had come up with another strategy for selling the ranch in case the Swiss investors' deal didn't go through, then saw a message from him that had come during the night while I slept:

I'm driving around and talking to government offices about a possible return back to Switzerland. It was very sad to see my kids and my granddaughter missing me. It looks now I may move back to Switzerland, where my roots are, sooner than later. Today I'm in Zurich. I'm just not a happy person in Arizona.

This message shot through my heart like an arrow. After I finished crying, I responded, "Does this mean you're leaving me?" I understood his desire to be with his children and grandchild and couldn't think of a better reason for him to leave me. I knew it was important that he be with his family for the remainder of his life.

Sitting on the steps outside the kitchen, watching the sunset, I saw an owl in the pine tree next to me begin barking like a dog. I looked to the right and saw two teenage-sized bobcats walking toward me just before they hopped up to the raised yard under the pine trees. I told them it was okay to come and drink water. When I stood up slowly, they turned around and ran away. I thought that was kind for the owl to warn me.

By October 15, my appetite was good. This was an indication that I was not in total decompensation. I seemed to be handling this better than previously in my life. Still, my heart was filled with great sorrow. I put all the objects in the backyard, garage, and patio as they were before I'd come, knowing I needed to start packing and making preparations to go to Durango. There was a man offering a free room in exchange for cooking for him. I had no other choice other than to be homeless. WhiteOne said they were arranging everything.

I waited another week. No message from Peter. I was beginning to understand that when he'd left on July 26, 2016, he was on a timeline where he left me and didn't return. The other Peter created in this decision was returning to me in Wickenburg, but I was not in that timeline. I was in the first timeline, where Peter returned, then went back to Switzerland. This was probably the convoluted universe, as Dolores Cannon discovered in her sessions. I focused on slowly packing up more objects that I would take with me to Colorado, cleaning the house, and preparing for Peter's temporary return. I just didn't know if I was to leave before he returned or afterward. We had agreed I would pick him up at the airport on the 26th of October, and I still intended to unless circumstances changed.

Focusing on Peter's children, grandchild, and their happiness was helping me to cope. My conscious mind wanted to focus on the what-ifs, but I just couldn't go there and stay there. I needed to stay present and healthy. I didn't feel I could talk to anyone but Virginia, yet I was not ready to talk with her either. I didn't want to end up crying on the phone, so I talked to the walls and the spirits that were there in the house. I talked with my angels and with the WhiteOne. I kept hearing their mantra as they repeated, "We love you very much."

On the 16th of October, I talked with Virginia, who agreed I needed to grieve because I was hearing Peter's voice more. He was talking with me about love as he had before. Virginia said, "How nice it was for you to greet him at his ascension." Then, the WhiteOne said this was what had occurred, and it was very beautiful. He was a little confused but instantly recognized me, so he was not lost along the way, and they had helped him to understand. He could now communicate with me in my mind. This reality was becoming so unlike anything I'd ever known before. Although I'd been introduced to these concepts, it was another thing to actually experience them.

On October 19, while talking with the WhiteOne, I mentioned that I thought it was an amazing concept to have souls coming and going out of the human vessels, especially for the ascension process. They said, "Well, dear Barbara, you're the one who helped us become informed of this concept in the first place because of the destruction-of-the-world research you've done. It is you who we thank. And this is why you are very curious about the backdrop person[28] concept. You specifically agreed and wanted to explore this concept firsthand so that we can further understand how the mind and heart can cope and process these interactions and feelings. It is a concept that is still being perfected."

On the 20th of October, I received a deep tissue massage from Nicolette. It had been four years since the last one. I brought extra napkins because I knew I would be crying. My left shoulder blade area was still inflamed and screaming in agony. When she started massaging, I felt immense pain on the left side. She worked on the left side of my back for a long time. Then, when Nicolette pressed hard on the right scapular area, where hard knotted muscles were located, I began to sob. And it came out big time. I cried and cried and cried. It was Peter.

---

28   Dolores Cannon coined the phrase "backdrop people" in her *Convoluted Universe Book IV*. These are people who look real, yet they are an image we see in the environment because so many have already ascended.

Nicolette dug deeper and helped me release the sorrow. When she massaged my left foot, it felt good. No pain, no tears. When she massaged the right foot, I went into an altered state and saw my life in review. Then, the life review centered on my current life with Peter, bringing all the memories forward. I released more sorrow, crying and crying. She and I were both surprised. Just about every part of my body was in pain where she touched except for the left foot. The psoas muscle and the gluteals were excruciatingly painful. My arms were even more intensely uncomfortable. My right hand even jumped in reflex, slightly hitting Nicolette's right upper arm. We both laughed as I apologized.

Then, it got downright hellish when she began massaging my neck. I thought I was going to pass out from the pain. Now at the neck, I was facing my truth. Facing my present. Facing my future. Facing my whole life. All the struggles, all the joys, and every single detail of my life seemed to be right there in my neck. Then she turned my head slightly to the right and began massaging the left side of the neck. I thought I was literally dying. I was in free fall inside the pain. Nobody could rescue me. I contemplated committing suicide by just leaving my body, but they wouldn't let me. I heard them. "You're doing good, dear one. Not many would face this as you have. Others would turn to alcohol, drugs, or a gunshot to stop it all. What we are about to tell you, you must not say to anyone until we deliver further information in your next QHHT® session. Do you understand? You will be married again, but not to Peter. This is part of the experience and the life lessons you are learning. And for this, we are grateful."

When the massage was finished, I released my overdistended bladder and then walked around in a daze. The endorphins were up at top level, flowing through my bloodstream, as was the cellular debris. The massive water intake began.

There was no message from Peter. No Skype. No phone call. Nothing. I needed to keep my critical judgment in check. I knew the new soul was playing his role. On a soul level, it must have been hard to have to cut me off. I sent more love to him and thanked him for his part in this experience. Then I was receiving more info about my move. I could put my stuff in storage there in Wickenburg, move half of my stuff in my SUV, return and get the rest, sleep in the hotel down the street if need be, and return to Colorado. At that point, I was just guessing if Peter was returning six days from now or not.

My mother left a message saying my dad had Alzheimer's disease and was going fast. I knew about Alzheimer's and that the person typically went through the stages very slowly, so I knew my mom wanted me to visit. I had been told to stay away and continue my personal inner work. This was very hard. Why did I have to go through this situation? I had four other siblings. It was not like I was the only one.

By October 23, my back started feeling better, though the soreness was still there. I packed up most of my stuff and planned to get up early the next day to get my vehicle into a repair shop for a tune-up to make sure she was roadworthy. I prayed to God the cost would be minimal. Each day was met with sorrow. I missed my Peter, the one who had kissed me every morning and every time he opened the door to his vehicle for me to sit on the passenger side. I cried and released as I taped up the boxes, knowing I would be living out of a suitcase for the next four to five months, trusting that God had plans for me and all would pass. In a way, I saw it as a hibernation time because it would be during the winter. I was hoping my clients would want angel card readings and channeled healing sessions because I could do that over the internet and phone.

On October 26, Peter arrived at Sky Harbor late that night, having had a cough for the last two weeks. He brought home European medicine, which he was taking. As we hugged in the airport, his energy was different and not just from a chest cold. This was not Peter. On the way home, he spoke in German. I thought he was talking in his sleep before he said he needed to pull over and urinate. I pulled over to the side of the road. After this brief pit stop, I drove us back to the ranch. Before we went to sleep at midnight, he told me in the kitchen that he had a girlfriend in Switzerland, and they'd been traveling together for the past month. He was not even living in the apartment in Aeschi. He'd almost turned around in the Los Angeles airport and boarded Flight 41 back to Zurich to be with her. He didn't want to be in America anymore—specifically in Arizona and especially with me.

How could this be happening? We didn't fight. We didn't argue during the summer while he was in Switzerland. I admit there was a change in him in the early summer. While driving during our errands in Phoenix, he'd said negative comments about other drivers. His foul attitude had begun getting on my nerves, and I'd asked him to try to be more positive about life. He'd yelled back at me, "Can't I say how I feel?" I'd replied, "If we focus on the negative, then that is what the universe will bring more of." We'd cherished every good connection over the internet and kept each other informed with email messages. There had been no mention of him not loving me anymore or asking me to change in some way. Had he been hiding his true feelings? I reminded myself that not everyone could talk about their feelings.

I felt like I was being shattered into a million pieces of broken glass on the floor. I did my qi gong and tai chi. My movements were fragile, unsteady, and off-balance as I wept. I felt detached from myself, unable to understand why this was happening. Everywhere I looked outdoors in the desert, I saw heart-shaped rocks. And when I bent over in the form, just below me was a hollowed-out hole in the soil in the shape of a heart. What was the message? Was my heart empty? Was it devoid of love and compassion? Was it a cleansing? Was it a message of Peter's love for me no longer being present? Was it a message of relocation? Answer: It was everything because it was all love.

He closed his office door so he could Skype with his new love in Switzerland. The food at breakfast that morning tasted awful, even though I'd placed my love in it. He didn't hold my hand during the blessing as before. He got up right after finishing the meal so he didn't have to spend one more second with me in his sight. I went to my bedroom to write the newsletter and journal this Earth walk of sorrow. Journaling provided an outlet for my emotions. I thanked God, my angels, my Higher Self, and Mother Earth for this experience. I knew it was part of my growth and the evolution of my soul. However, quite frankly, it sucked. No wonder souls don't want to come here to Earth, yet others do just so they can experience something like this. When you're in the middle of it, it's difficult. On the other side of it, you're relieved you made it through the pain.

I waited for Peter to ask me about my plans, figuring when he was ready to hear, he would ask. And so, at the end of lunch that day, he asked me when I was leaving. I told him my last client was the twelfth here in Wickenburg, I'd rented a trailer for the fourteenth, and I would be leaving the fifteenth. I asked if this was okay with him. He said yes. We needed to discuss the kitchen item distribution, and I told him I would leave the toaster and the coffee maker. When he was done using them, he could donate them to Habitat for Humanity. I would leave the microwave oven too. As the day drew near, I boxed up the knives, the Cuisinart blender, the food processor, and my baking tools.

It felt strange to not feel myself there fully, but rather like I was walking in a dream state, devoid of feelings of love and happiness. The wind blew hard that day. The external world was falling apart as I read about the elections, the corruption in government, the investigations, the Wikileaks announcements, etc., and so was my internal world. I felt like I was in a million pieces, shattered. However, there was an inner knowing that I would get to the other side of this. I would feel happiness and joy again someday. For now, the grieving must be walked through. I certainly didn't want to bury it and have it manifest illness in my body down the road. My heart remained open from this second-in-a-row blow to the heart. I thanked Peter and his new girlfriend for giving me this gift. We are all One, and I know we do these things for each other.

I was vigilant in looking for signs confirming this wasn't Peter, my Peter. After lunch, he put one of the steak knives in the dishwasher. Peter and I had agreed years ago that we would not do this because they could be dulled by the high-pressure water. He loved those knives. I was surprised. When he wasn't looking, I removed the knife from the dishwasher and handwashed it.

This soul was spending hours on Skype behind his closed office door, talking with a woman in German. The sound of their voices carried through the door as I put on my sneakers in the adjacent room. I was a little perturbed because he was talking for hours, and she was not encouraging him to drink extra water. He came out thirsty, and the fact that he was taking Dextromethorphan to bring up the mucus in his chest was troubling to me as a former nurse, and I still loved him. It didn't matter to me that he was another soul. I still loved and cared for him as I did Peter.

I continued to observe. When we had our afternoon milk-coffee and homemade pumpkin bread, he faced away from me on the other side of the kitchen. The message was clear. I was not wanted nor needed in his life. He didn't ask me for help anymore. Why was I being so civil? Why did I care? It was because I understood from a higher perspective that we all play roles for each other. We have contracts and agreements with one another. This situation was giving me the opportunity to walk through it without drama.

By the end of October, I'd found more data points that this was not the Peter I knew before. For the past eight years, my bananas were kept next to the knives. Peter's bananas were on the opposite side of the counter, near the door. He liked his bananas riper than I do. He ate both of my bananas and didn't touch his.

I told Peter in my mind, *"Show me evidence that you are here and are ascended. Give me the sign or whatever, and make it so it is very easy to see and recognize."*

In the morning, Pete killed a rattlesnake. I walked over to the vulture plate (an area of poured concrete where we leave food scraps for the animals) and saw it was moving its tail slightly. Pete said that it was just nerves. I thought it was still alive, so I kept my distance. Later that day, my dear friend Rose drove up to Wickenburg in her new truck, and we went out to lunch. When Rose and I returned, I stepped out of her truck, walked toward the front entry staircase, and saw a rattlesnake curled up asleep at the bottom step.

I went inside and told Pete to get his snake pole. He came out and killed the snake. We looked, and there was no dead snake on the vulture plate. We saw tracks. It was obvious the snake had moved from the concrete plate to the staircase. I saw that Peter was telling me he was still there, and the staircase represented the ascension. The fact that the snake did not die was Peter telling me he was still alive on the other side. I spoke with Lance later, and he added that Pete would be releasing something really big for him. The snake was the toxins, the old programs, and the old patterns. They were also releasing from me, and my next relationship would be extremely awesome.

The next morning (October 31), as I woke up, I received more info from the WhiteOne. The snake was Peter's message to me, letting me know he had walked out and into the body and had ascended. The snake impression in the gravel from the concrete plate to the staircase showed a single line, then there was a portion where two snake lines ran parallel to one another, then it went back into one line impression. I found it interesting that the snake (Peter) stopped at the stairs because the staircase represented ascension. Peter didn't die, and this was why I could hear him. I then noticed that the snake was sleeping, meaning that Peter was resting on the other side. I had asked him the day before to give me a sign that he was with me and ascended—a sign that was very easy to see, hard to miss, not too over-the-top, yet something I would know was him. The snake had provided the message. A rattle-snake provokes one's attention like no other symbol.

November 1, I stood in the kitchen with Pete, looking at his body. I wanted so much to run into his arms and be held. I couldn't. He was not Peter. It felt so odd that I couldn't be with him like I'd been for the past eight years. I understood I must respect and honor this new soul and was grateful he was able to communicate with me and not act in a fashion that was unbearable. I wanted so much to tell him that I knew who he was and was okay with it. What I found fascinating was that we, who are close to our loved ones, are not cognizant of the agree-ments souls have made. We just have to figure it out ourselves. Was I stepping into new territory?

On the 8th of November, I woke up feeling at ease when I saw that Donald Trump had won the election. I felt there was hope, and we would thrive once more. At 10:00 a.m., I drove over to Nicolette's and received a deep tissue massage. We found the left gluteals were completely released, but my upper back and neck had quite a bit of knotting. The right gluteals were extremely tense. My legs felt won-derful. There was some burning in the left lower inner thigh area. The right hand, between the thumb and index finger at the base, had a very tender area. When she worked on my left mid-back and the neck areas, there were times I could not breathe. The pain was very intense. We did good work. I cried a lot and released.

I sat outside the next day and enjoyed the breeze. I had an inner knowing that all would be well. It was just the transition that was the hardest, like breaking through into the new—the unfamiliar—that was out of our comfort zone. I ate my breakfast by myself that morning because Pete was talking with his girlfriend. At least he was feeling better and recovering from his bronchitis. I was grateful for this.

The next day, I woke up at 5:00 a.m. with increased energy, and my muscles felt good. I packed up my SUV and placed everything but my clothes in the garage. I was praying that everything would fit in the cargo trailer, and I would be able to pack it properly and safely without hurting myself. I walked out to the promontory point outside the ranch, to the place where we had permission from the neighbors to walk. I blessed the land and all inhabitants and gave my gratitude to God and Mother Earth. I said goodbye to the fairies, the horse, and the sheep spirits. I prayed for strength to drive safely and deliberately toward Durango. I asked for the most powerful angels to be by my side, assisting in a smooth and easy drive up there. I said goodbye to Grandfather Pine and the trees, the rock people, the plant people, and to this life on the ranch. I did my Kriya Yoga for the last time in Arizona, followed by an Epsom salt bath soak.

It was the 14th of November when I picked up the U-Haul cargo trailer. All the way home, I worried that the trailer would not be big enough. WhiteOne responded to my concerns each time that it was big enough. After loading it up, I saw they were right. It was such an optical illusion when you didn't see everything stacked up inside the trailer. I fell down on my right knee, and my low back had a little discomfort, so I applied ice on my back and knee, soaking it in Epsom salts again. I burst into tears while packing the trailer, let it release, and felt better. The trip started at 5:00 a.m. the next day.

I woke up at 3:33 a.m. after a rough night fighting with my ego that wanted to worry about the drive. As I walked to the door, Peter came into the kitchen and said, "Well, I hope you have success in your new adventures. Who knows, you may be famous, and I'll see you on the news." I could not respond to this. I didn't know what to say or what it meant. He hugged me goodbye, and there was nothing there. A human body with a soul who came to perform the task. It could be very well that the soul left as soon as I pulled out of the ranch. I looked at my watch as I pulled out in front of the garage: 5:15 a.m.

I cried all the way to Durango. The drive did not feel good. Not like in 2009 when we vacationed for nine days through Colorado, Utah, and Arizona. I arrived at Virginia's place at 5:15 p.m., exactly twelve hours from when I'd left the ranch. I didn't feel comfortable there. I was beyond exhaustion, and my headache was so severe that I could hardly eat the wonderful food Virginia prepared for my little supper. I slept in their home office on an inflatable bed. I had a hard time sleeping, crying for my Peter. Once again, I found myself totally out of my comfort zone. My energy systems were fried.

The next morning, I cried at breakfast. Virginia drove ahead of me as we went to Frank's home. It was a gracious meeting; however, when I first saw him, I got an intuitive hit in two seconds that something was not right. The realization struck me like a semitruck. I reminded myself that I must see how this all would play out.

CHAPTER 11

Winter in Durango: My Soul's Darkest Night

T HE HOME WAS NICE AND very clean because a housekeeper came in once a week. The neighborhood was set in a forest with beautiful ponds and streams running through it. My headache felt awful. I thought I had altitude sickness. For some reason, I looked up instead of down and fell down the garage stairs, spraining my right ankle. Virginia came over and helped us empty the car and place my stuff in the art studio next to the garage. The trailer was emptied. I then took the trailer to the local U-Haul rental center down the road, all with a screaming sprained ankle.

I found out quickly that people in Durango have two or three jobs because they couldn't afford the high cost of living. There was no middle class. You were either dirt poor or very wealthy.

Feeling awful with this headache and nausea, I could barely eat. I ended up resting on the sofa with ice on my right foot, sleeping and listening to Frank talk. He enjoyed my stories. Now, I understood why Virginia's Higher Self wanted me to get up to Durango as soon as possible. Two days after my arrival, the first snow fell. Last night was just yucky with the headache and nausea all night long. I kept crying. I was constantly thirsty and drank water all night long.

On November 18, I woke up feeling much better and regained my appetite since the headache had disappeared. My energy was increasing. I spent a good part of the day organizing my stuff in the studio, then later spoke with my friend, Diana, in Phoenix. She recommended I take my porcelain dolls inside. I did get a little tired in the afternoon, so I rested a bit on the sofa. My foot was 99 percent healed, and the bruising was almost gone, so I did some active range of motion exercises with my right foot.

As the day went on, I sorted through my emails, put a lot into the trash, and answered some. I spoke with Lance today. He said I sounded much better and agreed what I'd gone through was like going to another planet. This transition was more difficult than I'd anticipated. My head was clearer, and I was almost ready to accept new clients. I was preparing to cook more, but I needed to organize the kitchen. The pantry was a mess. Little by little, I created my new reality. I made a green smoothie with spinach, and Frank enjoyed it. The fog of my depression and grief began to lift. When I looked at the tree branches devoid of leaves, it reminded me of myself, like all my joy was stripped away. My reference point was stripped. My familiar was stripped.

Something very odd happened on the 23rd of November. I gave Frank a channeled healing session in the house, and this was the first time I observed a client burping nonstop for a full hour. His left face twitched almost nonstop too. He told me he felt he was moving energy. When I checked in to make sure he was okay, he said he was. He kept clearing his throat, then began jerking his head and upper shoulders like someone was knocking him around on the bed. I stood there watching this after I completed the right leg work and was no longer touching his body. The Higher Self worked on his brain, his heart, and his solar plexus chakra. I saw his ET form during the healing session. When he came out, I told him to take his time getting up, gave him a glass of water, and reminded him to drink extra water for the next seven days. He forgets things easily, and I noticed he didn't lay with his head straight and centered. After the session, instead of resting and letting the energies integrate as I recommended, he was flying around the house doing paperwork. After supper, when I prepared the kitchen for the Thanksgiving meal the next day, he hung out in the kitchen asking what I was doing. He seemed to be a bit intimidated by the kitchen and food preparation and followed me around like a puppy dog. There were times when he stood very close to me, and when I moved to give myself space, he moved toward me, not respecting boundaries. This behavior was not making sense to me.

November 24, 2016, while reading a screenplay written by a friend, I heard Frank's body jerking in his recliner. I looked over and watched him twitch as his right hand was weaving. I asked him about what was happening, and he told me he was releasing his blocks to compassion and patience. I received a download, "His healing is continuing." I told him that occasionally, it takes time for healing to complete. We checked in with each other about our activities and plans. The crockpot made a wonderful pot roast. I added cucumber salad and a carrot salad and made smoothies to enjoy that evening. Frank said he enjoyed the meal, then went for a walk shortly before the roast was ready. I waited a half hour, then decided to eat by myself. Following my inner guidance, my body's needs, I ate by myself and gave a blessing of gratitude for everything.

I did my qi gong and tai chi outdoors the next day, still getting winded from the altitude. My legs were a bit wobbly, and I hoped the muscles would increase in strength as I continued to practice every other day. My Expedition's heater was not working, so I found a car repair shop and scheduled an appointment.

Before the night was over, I discovered all but one email that Peter had sent me was gone from my email program. I'd had a headache during the night, likely due to too much physical activity by walking to a restaurant for lunch while the car repair was done. I had to drink water several times through the night, then had to urinate many times. I felt depressed again. Everything I did or looked at reminded me of Peter and the eight years we'd spent together at the ranch. The WhiteOne reminded me they love me and would help me. Wanting more healing clients and angel tarot card reading clients, I asked for assistance so the money energy would go into my accounts and I could remain thriving and responsible for paying my bills on time. I reminded myself to be grateful for where I was and what had been provided for me. During the night, I had a realization that I didn't care whether I lived or died. It was an interesting place to be. My ego refused to believe this had happened. I still felt unsettled, as if I was out on a small boat, no oars, just drifting on the open sea, alone.

There had been no message about my father. There were moments when I felt I'd truly gone insane. I was sitting there out of my comfort zone, feeling alone, trying to get a firm grasp of a reference point that felt comforting. It was just not there. Why was the comfort out of my reach? The only place I was finding comfort was within, with God. During qi gong that next afternoon, I felt peace. Just like in 2008, before I moved out of my home in Peoria, it was qi gong and tai chi that helped me process the mental and emotional stress.

It snowed the next night. I did my qi gong and tai chi in the snow that morning while the pumpkins cooked in the oven. After tai chi, I did drunken master, then swan, then horse stance. That's when my body heated up so much that I had to take off my winter outerwear: coat, alpaca hat, gloves, and warm scarf. Practicing tai chi and qi gong with winter clothes was like being inside of a marshmallow. I told Zeysan that in a phone conversation, and he laughed. The high-altitude pumpkin bread I made came out tasting delicious.

Upon inquiry, I discovered Frank was channeling and didn't know it. He talked out loud, in a mumbling manner, asking questions and receiving answers. He shared with me that he didn't "fit in" with the neighbors of this community, that he felt different because they weren't awake. It was obvious to me that the Higher Self wanted me to get up to Colorado before the snow came, and it was obvious that they wanted me to be there for Frank's soul's transition from this Earthly existence. He was doing a lot of clearing every day through sinus drainage and belching large amounts of air.

Around 4:00 p.m., I felt an emptiness inside and felt so far away from my life that I couldn't even recognize who or where I was. It was not that I was ungrateful for everything, just that I was not feeling grounded and happy. My life in Arizona seemed so far away. I missed the people in my life. This ascension process was not an easy one to experience. I felt depressed and looked forward to sleep because I could leave my body and didn't have to be there. This must be why excessive sleeping is a component of depression. I needed to be more productive in the other realms while I slept. The WhiteOne said I would be there in this home with Frank for five months, so I asked, "Then what?" No answer.

By December 6, I was still crying over Peter and the abrupt change in my life, though still trying hard to be calm and centered. The memories kept returning. I sent a text message to Lance that said, "This grief thing sucks!" But my phone showed it as not delivered. Within forty-five seconds, Lance called me. He got the message in his mind to call me. We had a good laugh about the telepathy between us. I was one of the many souls he was helping in this lifetime, and I was very glad to have him give counsel during this experience.

I walked to the mailbox at the entrance to the neighborhood in the snow with my snow boots. I tried the attached hat for my coat, and it worked wonderfully. It kept my entire head and ears warm. I consider this goose down coat a wise investment, and it was proving itself so.

When the Snake Fist DVD arrived, I watched the beginning and began the form outdoors after my qi gong and tai chi. I did just the very first move slowly several times. I made it to almost 6:00 p.m. without crying. During a movie I watched on YouTube, there was a commercial for Swiss airlines three times. I patiently waited for my Colorado registration approval so I could facilitate QHHT® sessions. In the meantime, I continued to write my QHHT® session stories book and cook. I turned on the humidifier in my room to increase the moisture. I still had to get up two times that night to urinate and drink water. However, the thirst response was gone. This meant I was keeping up with my body's fluid levels.

Virginia and I met for lunch and walked to the office. Walking through the practitioner's front office, I was shocked at the mess and dust. By the time we reached the QHHT® office located in the back, I was in a daze. When I entered the QHHT® section of the office, I heard clairaudiently, "Welcome, welcome, we've been waiting for you." We sat for a bit and talked about logistics and fees. I was still not clear how this shared business arrangement would be worked out.

On December 23, 2016, I wrote to Hoyt and wished him Merry Christmas. I just wanted to connect with another human I knew. He wrote back and told me about his medical journey. His heart surgery had gone well, and his doctors were pleased. He went to Casa Grande, Arizona, for a Christmas dinner with a sister he had never met. Hoyt's father had married many times and fathered many children. I sat there wishing I could help Hoyt clean the house and make it easier for him to recuperate. To care for the cats. How did life turn out like that? I told Hoyt I was living in Durango, waiting to work, and had left by myself. He didn't ask about the circumstances.

I ordered a camp stove from the online REI store, the one I'd been looking at for the past year and a half. I bought it partly for preparedness, in case the electricity was cut off due to a storm or an electric grid interruption. At least I'd be able to boil water for food preparation. I also purchased it partly for camping. Now, I just needed to buy the propane canisters at Walmart. I couldn't depend upon Frank for emergency tasks because he just didn't know what to do, nor was he able to handle a tough situation. I didn't think he had any basic life skills. My Higher Self told me not to worry and that we'd be taken care of always.

I began the new year noticing that Frank was belching more frequently and at a louder volume, all day and all night. The sounds were sickening to me. I suggested he see his doctor. Frank kept having meltdowns, getting easily overwhelmed about things in his life. My Higher Self was telling me to focus on my life, not his. He went in and out of this reality, sometimes saying he didn't hear me when I asked a question. He only partially heard what I said. Lance taught me to just be quiet and watch what happens. Sure enough, Frank would answer the question after I was quiet. This was the person coming back into reality, and the Higher Self answered the question. I found this phenomenon fascinating.

Last week while driving in the neighborhood, I saw Frank walking away from the house. I saw his side view, distinct clothing, and gait and was certain it was him. When I walked into the house and down the hallway about two minutes later, he was in his bedroom. I asked him if he had gone for a walk. He said he had in the morning, but it was at the recreation center in town, and he drove his car there. I asked the neighbor across the street if there was another man in the neighborhood that looked and walked like him. The neighbor said no. What may have happened was an interface with two dimensions, two timelines, or I saw Frank in a parallel life.

As I was preparing lunch, adding more vegetables to the menu on

Wednesday, Frank came into the kitchen and asked me when lunch would be ready. I said in an hour. He started giving me a hard time about eating his own deli food. I told him he could do whatever he wanted, either eat his deli food or wait till lunch was ready. He jumped on me, saying he's just trying to get along. I told him it was his decision. He then said he was having a bad day. I told him this didn't give him the right to take it out on me. I was not his punching bag. It was not my fault that he hadn't done anything like going to a medical doctor before I came last November, and I reminded him again that he needed to see a doctor. Frank started washing the dishes while I was cooking, so I asked him to please do the dishes after I finished cooking. He got mad and said no one was there, so he was washing the dishes. I told him, "That's not true. I am here, and I am using the kitchen to cook."

On February 18, 2017, I walked out to the studio where my boxes were located and cried because I missed Peter very much and over what it took to get me to leave Arizona. I needed to look at it and see it as a gift of love that I gave myself. In the meantime, nothing was making sense to me. I no longer had gas money to go to the office. Obviously, the WhiteOne wanted me out of the office. I thought I'd reached rock bottom and there was no further descent, then this occurred. While this was not in alignment with my belief in placing our energy into the space, we did agree I must surrender. My Higher Self wanted me focused on the QHHT® session stories book. Virginia wondered if I was to be at the house for some reason that concerned Frank. We didn't know, so we observed.

The snow began to melt at the end of February. I walked through the woods every day for peace, quiet, and healing, being mindful of bears. The neighbors had taught me how to recognize bear tracks and evidence of their presence in the environment. There were bears that walked around the neighborhood. I was now eating my meals in my room because Frank wanted to argue at the dining table. I couldn't accept any more of his confrontational behavior. I didn't want to be in this house anymore, but I had to. I redirected my energy and focused on my work.

As time progressed, Frank's anger escalated. He tried to verbally lash out at me whenever we were in the same room. I wondered if he could benefit from mental therapy and recommended this help to him, but he wouldn't go. My guides were telling me to stay away from him as much as possible. I was told not to talk with him because anything I said would be twisted around to start an argument. I did a forgiveness tapping for myself regarding Frank. He'd taught me a lot those past three months. I'd never lived with anyone who didn't have life skills. I found out that the person who lived there six months before I did had used the studio as an office, and that's where she hung out. The rest of the time, she was at her place of work or out with friends.

During the night of March 4, Frank's spirit came into my room in an etheric manner. It was about two in the morning. I sat up and asked, "What is going on?" My Higher Self removed him. I didn't understand why he would want to come into my room. His constant belching and mumbling was really getting on my nerves. I kept busy doing my work and focusing on getting out of this home.

On March 6, I met with Virginia in the afternoon for a discussion at her other office. She shared with me that all she had left in funds was one more month to pay the rent for the QHHT® office. I shared that with the marketing I'd been doing, going out in the community and placing advertisements in the businesses. It wasn't enough. She had spent a considerable amount of money on advertisements in a local holistic magazine. We placed a sign in the window of the office for people to see as they drove by on Highway 550 toward town. It still wasn't enough.

I told her I was really having a difficult time processing Frank's behaviors, then I broke down and cried. Virginia said this was the PhD of human experiences. She told me that she thought as a nurse, I would have more compassion. I told her it's totally different being a nurse in the hospital where you can go home and take a break from it. Frank's constant belching and mumbling was causing constant stress. I had to walk to the woods every day just to find peace. Virginia asked if I would go into hypnosis with her. I agreed, and we went up to the office. Virginia didn't like the answers from my Higher Self. She was disappointed with the platitudes. This meant she had expectations, even though I'd told her we should go into this session without ex-pectations, no matter what the answers were. My Higher Self refused to give her more information. There must have been a reason for this. The WhiteOne did show me a scene from my future when Frank and I are on the other side, in spirit, sitting on a park bench. We give each other a high five hand slap, congratulating ourselves for the project we worked on together to make me stronger.

Then I got it! This whole experience in Colorado was a strengthening one. This was the design of the dark night of the soul experience.

I started emotional freedom tapping to change my perception of Frank. On the 8th of March, I noticed a very different personality. He was happy and whistling. I asked WhiteOne if there was a soul swap. They said that yes, Frank ascended.

It was Friday, the 10th of March, when the housekeeper walked into the house and Frank spoke with her, very happy and friendly. The housekeeper had a perplexed look on her face and asked, "Who was that?" When I walked down the hall with her, and she saw his bedroom sliding glass door blinds wide open, she gasped and took a step backward. "Oh my God!" She'd never seen them open, and she had been there longer than I had. I could feel his energy was different. It was lighter, and I could converse in a friendly way with this new soul. I was now wondering if this soul would live longer in Frank's body.

On the 13th of March, I was looking forward to my future. Even though my heart was wanting love, it also wanted to go home. Not to Source or another planet. My heart wanted to be in a loving relationship again, but I was not ready. I had more work to do on myself.

On the fifteenth, I heard this message from The WhiteOne: "Your mission here at the house is complete. The next phase of your journey here begins. Your mission was to help Frank ascend. Just like you helped Peter to ascend. You're now becoming familiar with this work of yours."

Yesterday, after months of recommending he go to the urgent care clinic down the road where doctors were available for his sinus problems, he walked into the kitchen and announced, "Thank you for suggesting I go to the urgent care. I saw a doctor, and they took a sample for testing. They gave me a doctor to go to."

I was doing more emotional freedom tapping and feeling better. I did a little bit of crying and releasing yesterday too. At noon, I walked into the Sacred Space store in Durango and met the owner, Melissa, and her lovely employee, Savannah. After four hours of talking and receiving messages and sharing confirmation, Melissa wanted a QHHT® session. I also met Bodhi, her dog, who was an amazing being. He responded positively to my energy. Later that week, Melissa arrived at the office with Bodhi. He rolled around on the floor, expressing his joy and excitement. We began the interview, and Bodhi settled down. We practitioners invite our client's pets to join us in sessions. They love the energies and receive healing too. This was a particularly fascinating QHHT® session for me to facilitate because of the information revealed.

From hard physical work, Melissa had sustained a ruptured disc and fractured vertebra in her lower spine. Although she'd had surgery for the injury, for several years, she had been complaining of continued alternating intermittent leg pain. Her doctors thought she was just seeking attention. She met an angel of a man who connected her with a world-renowned neurosurgeon, and he was flabbergasted upon viewing her lower spinal magnetic resonance imaging film that she was able to walk at all. The neurosurgeon conducted a twelve-hour surgery involving the spinal nerves and bones. Melissa came out of the recovery phase in the most intense pain. It was so much, it sent her out of her mind. If you read the first chapter of my autobiography, where I described the excruciating pain that caused me to grab equipment and supplies without restraint or control, screaming obscenities at everyone in earshot, you would understand the degree of Melissa's suffering. In other words, that much pain can absolutely cause a person to go completely bonkers.

During her hospitalization in the neurological intensive care unit, Melissa had to be tied down with restraints to keep the life-sustaining equipment on and in her for her benefit. She said a nurse stayed at her bedside, refused to leave her, and the nurse looked like me. The nurse asked her about her children because Melissa could not remember she had two sons. As Melissa came into consciousness and realized she had children, the nurse kept talking with her, helping her to calm down and be still. She made a full recovery. Melissa felt the nurse who had cared for her saved her life. Three months prior to this session, a dear friend mentioned to Melissa that she had said out loud, "I wish I could meet that nurse who saved my life in critical care." When Melissa first saw me, she knew without a doubt I was that nurse. She was hesitant to tell me because she did not want to shock me. She waited until her private QHHT® session with me to reveal I was the nurse who saved her life.

Melissa was very intuitive and extremely accurate with her psychic skills, to the point that those connected and in communication with the star beings from other places in the universe and planes of existence respect and revere her.

Melissa and I spoke the next day, and she gave me a small amount of the transmission of information. Her voice was excited, and she was adamant that I be informed of the information she was holding. We agreed for her to give me a reading in her office.

Brenda, my client from Oregon, had a wonderful QHHT® session. She was very intuitive. Brenda could feel the negative energy of the front office and the contrast to the loving, high vibration of the inner QHHT® office without me saying anything. Later, she gifted me with a birthday card. Brenda made it with one of her beautiful sunset photos. It touched me deeply. I cried because of the many sunsets Peter and I used to watch at the ranch, sitting on the steps outside the kitchen.

On March 30, when I went out to the garage and pushed the garage door opener button, the spring broke. The garage door was stuck shut. I asked Frank to call the service out to fix it, but he told me he didn't know who to call. I suggested he call the number on the garage door, but that number didn't work. I recommended he look up a repair service in the phonebook. He refused to look up a garage door repair service because his mind was too messed up. I asked him how this was different than any other day. He said it was worse today. I called the service and was told a repairman was in the neighborhood and would come by in about two hours. We were blessed.

I had a reading with Melissa that afternoon, and it was amazing. Bodhi greeted me with kindness, love, and respect. Melissa mentioned I needed to read the book, *Blue Star*, write a letter to my guides/Higher Self, and be specific about what I wanted. I was to understand that there are multiple entities occupying Frank's body, and they were

messing with me. I needed to tell Frank I am a loving and compassionate soul and that his energy and behaviors were hurting my heart. Melissa said I was leaving Frank's home at the end of April or sooner and
that Virginia and I were done with the QHHT® office arrangement. She
gave me confirmation of information I already knew but didn't want
to totally admit. We humans want the best and for things to work out.
Sometimes, we just need to get out of our own way. God has plans. If
God wanted me there, I would be there. If God wanted me someplace
else, I'd be someplace else. I remind myself, but for the grace of God,
go I.

I purchased a dream interpretation by Lance and called him to talk
about the white cat with the arrow in its body walking toward me. The
buildings were white. I called the vet and was in the process of making
preparations for emergency care of the cat. A woman was surprised
that I was helping the cat. Lance said the cat was me, and the part of
it that was attacked by energy was a part of me that needed healing.
With his guidance, I called the light of God into me through my crown
chakra, down into my heart, and out through my hands, sending the
healing love energy to the kitty. I watched the arrow move out of the
kitty, and the kitty was healed. The kitty jumped up on my lap as my
lower legs shook. Lance could hear the popping in the room he was in
at the same time, confirmation of the release.

On the last day of March, when the cleaning woman showed up at
the house, Frank was flitting around like a butterfly talking with her,
making decisions about how to wash his comforter. He was engaging
with her, acting like a "normal" person. I was observing his changing
personality from one day to the next, realizing he was acting like there
was no meltdown mode.

I received a message from my Higher Self, through my feelings, to
start packing my spices and kitchen utensils because this was the last
meal I was cooking. While walking down the hall, I passed by Frank's
office and then stood in the hallway, at the wide-open double French
doors. There on his desk, I saw the copy of my autobiography that I
had given him to read. On top of my book was another book entitled,
Dark Night of the Soul. I shook my head and said to myself and the

universe, "Very funny. You have quite the sense of humor. Message received!"

In the beginning of April, I perceived Virginia and I were not in sync regarding the QHHT® office. It appeared we were in separate worlds. I sat for a minute and asked myself what was going on there? This was messaging between Virginia and myself that I really needed to be on my own. We needed to part ways. Business partnership-type relationships are not for everyone. I now understood my mission in Durango was more about the ascension work. Durango was too small of a town to support a steady service of people who wanted regression hypnosis for healing.

It was also becoming evident that I must move my items in the art studio into a storage unit until I knew where to go next. I was in the moment, observing, hour by hour. I'd decided to rent a storage unit in Hermosa, less than a mile from me, until I figured out where to go. I told myself that I was walking through a normal progression on my path. There was no drama but a forward movement. I spoke with my friend Rose, in Phoenix, who had felt the intuition to call me. She said she could feel me. I gave her the gist of the story, and she agreed something was coming so I could leave.

That evening, I asked WhiteOne if there was anything I hadn't done, commanded, or asked for? They said no, I'd done everything.

I then said out loud, "I am giving all of what I am experiencing right now to you, dear God, and allowing you to give me the best and greatest outcome. I also put in the same request for Melissa."

They replied, "Yes, very much so."

I then looked at my phone. It was 7:07 p.m. The 707 message was, "God's wisdom was guiding you in the right way. Move forward with confidence." *Thank you, God!*

During the night of the 7th of April, I experienced intense energies. My brain was pulsating. The WhiteOne said it was a mass ascension of 5 percent more of the Durango population. That meant 95 percent of the population had ascended. I didn't know the exact figures. I just trusted that all was being taken care of. I received information to ask Hoyt if I could stay in the guest room of his home until I found a place on my own. I sent Hoyt an email message conveying my request and offered to help clean up his house and do light home maintenance.

He wrote, "Sure."

I felt a huge release of tension. An energy shift occurred. My vibration began to soar. And now, with that release, I was able to feel the negative dense energies in Frank's house even more. I kept my mind busy with the moving tasks. This action brought me peace as the forward movement was engaged. It felt like I was going home to Arizona. I was full circle, yet stronger and perceiving life in a larger way. I was grateful. I was very grateful to tears to be of help to Hoyt, even if it was for only a little while. I prayed to God to let him be healthy and asked for a safe journey back to Phoenix.

I tell my clients we must take action and then God puts into place what we desire and need. We can't just sit in our home and think something magical will happen. We must take action because this is God taking action.

Yesterday, when I opened the kitchen blinds in the early evening, six deer were walking to the house and grazing on the grass. I knew this was a good sign of forward movement, breaking into the new.

The tears turned more to gratitude than sorrow. I had come to Durango to process. I cried every day, most of the time waking up in the middle of the night, processing the blow to the heart known as abandonment. Being in this vortex of energy caused the processing to be experienced at lightning speed, Godspeed. Dear Melissa had been so kind checking in on me as I emerged from this dark night of the soul. She called me every day.

I requested a change of address with the postal office via the internet and deferred my cell phone bill until the next month. I was asking God to make sure the money was there for everything at the right moment, in divine timing, and being reassured that it would all work out. Virginia had cautioned me that if I were to move out of Frank's home, I would need to do it quickly because there could be sabotage, meaning Frank would come up with an excuse for me not to go. Whether it was conscious or unconscious, it could happen. I took those wise words into consideration. I planned to stay at the Hampton Inn hotel in Durango the night before I left.

On the 11th of April, during my walk into the woods, I came to the realization that God was playing with God. That's what was really going on. The negative was all part of the game, as well as the positive. Nineteen more days before I left Colorado, and my energy increased. I felt lighter and happier. I understood that the past five months of experience had strengthened me. I was going to Arizona, and I walked with trust, faith, and confidence I would be provided for and prosper. I walked in the dark, trusting that God had better plans for me. I walked to the Animas River and channeled the mathematical star language, allowing the energies to flow through the body movement of my arms, hands, and fingers. Two Canadian geese flew over me, and I saw four small spring green snakes on my walk, sunning in the afternoon warmth of the dirt trail.

On the 23rd of April, I channeled the WhiteOne for the Star Energy Healing Teleconference. Star codes were adjusted. Powerful healing occurred, and they had me guide the participants with the star tetrahedron.

My plan had been to walk out the door and not look back on Sunday, May 7, 2017.

I would write my books, and they would be published. I would become a certified hypnotherapist. Dolores Cannon was encouraging me to do so.

Another neighbor told me that the woman who had lived there for the six months before I came had aged ten years in that span of time. Clearly, Frank's inappropriate behavior had been experienced by others. It wasn't just me. With greater clarity, I understood he provided strengthening growth for all who interacted with him. Still, it was a difficult process to experience.

By the 2nd of May, the storage unit was packed, the U-Haul trailer was arranged, and I'd decided where to eat breakfast the morning of my departure from the house. I was sitting there at my desk, asking myself, "This is my life?" I asked my Higher Self, "What do I do now?" I'd thought of everything. I'd prepared everything, and I'd done everything. I'd already talked with my friends. There was no one to call. The belching, moaning, and groaning continued. Now what? I heard, "Relax and watch a movie."

Unfortunately, my family still wanted to put me in a straightjacket and throw me in an asylum because of my spiritual healing gifts. Their communications via voicemail messages were hateful, and my mother had been sending me hateful birthday cards and messages for the past three years. With each card, I held it in my hands and sent love and compassion to her. I did not judge my mother because I knew it must be very painful for her. In my mind and heart, I knew this was a life lesson project my mother and I were working on.

On May 7, I walked out of the house at 7:00 a.m., having left a letter for Frank on the bedroom dresser. I forgave him and asked him to forgive me. I thanked him and wished him the best in life. I had breakfast at the Hermosa Grill, then picked up the cargo trailer. It took me four hours to fill it. I ate my lunch at the Hermosa Grill too. Everyone was so nice and courteous to me. After I finished my lunch and checked into the Hampton Inn, it felt good to get settled into the room. I slept very well that night. I was grateful to tears that there was no more belching, vomiting, moaning, and groaning sounds coming from the next room! The silence felt wonderful! The energy felt neutral.

No surprise, I was first in line for breakfast in the morning. This was the behavior of a highly motivated individual. It felt so good to see the horizon, the vast desert views, and the blue skies as I drove out of the area. I felt free for the first time in five months. Climbing out of the Animas Valley felt like a rebirthing experience in meditation work. A heavy weight was lifted off my shoulders. This was a physical experience. I could literally breathe freely and effortlessly. I drove from Durango to Glendale, Arizona, in ten and a half hours. My vehicle did well. I was grateful the dark night of my soul was over. But was it?

CHAPTER 12

Return to Arizona and My Family

I ARRIVED AT HOYT'S AT SIX in the evening and found the house in a disaster state. Cat urine and feces covered the floors, along with vomit, cat hair, bougainvillea leaves, and debris throughout the entire house. Hoyt had developed cellulitis the day after I'd asked to stay at his place and had to elevate his left leg instead of cleaning the house as he'd intended. Upon my examination, it was swollen and peeling, and the skin was darkened. He was on a course of antibiotics and could only manage to take cat naps and eat minimal food. He told me he had no money since his employer put him on a part-time basis, but he was looking for more work. I found all of this very upsetting, but at the same time, I knew this would pass.

While Hoyt watched TV, I cleaned the one kitchen countertop just to have somewhere to prepare food that was sanitary. He was shocked at the clean countertop and told me he was unaware there was cat poop all over the house. I knew he was color blind, but the smell was overwhelming. I could hardly breathe in the house, even with all the windows and doors open. The twenty-plus cats didn't even sleep in the house anymore because they had turned it into a huge litter box. There were cats in the house eating food. There were cats on the patio, in the backyard, and on the roof. The home remodel we had done twenty-three years before while married was all ruined. At least I had been able to enjoy it for the first eleven years. It was heartbreaking to look at the destruction. All of our photos still hanging on the walls made it all the more devastating somehow.

The ammonia level in the house affected my brain. I became upset and contemplated suicide for about five minutes. I knew I couldn't stay there, but I had nowhere else to go. When I laid down on the bed and closed my eyes that first night, my third eye opened, and I saw faces of people surrounding me. I thanked them, but I told them that they must leave. I sent them into the light, then cried myself to sleep and slept horribly.

The next day, I woke up to the continued nightmare. After breakfast, I took the cargo trailer back to U-Haul and rented one of their climate-controlled storage units to put most of my belongings in since I couldn't store anything at Hoyt's. He had hoarded massive quantities of garbage, cat excrement, papers, boxes, and indescribable junk. When I'd met him years before, the garage had been filled with boxes, tools, and debris, and only his motorcycle could fit in there. It was as if he'd reverted back to before I met him. The house was in order, but the garage wasn't. It took three hours and a whole lot of water consumption to empty the trailer and the car. I prayed, "God, please get me out of here now. I am willing to move on to the next part of the story. I know you have plans for me. Wherever you want me to go, I will go." I knew I didn't need to fix anything there for Hoyt. He had charted his course. He was an adult and knew better than to live in such squalor.

Without an appetite, I ate a sandwich, then went to the credit union to talk with Gloria, my financial angel. She came out of her office cubicle and hugged me. When I told her about Hoyt's home, she shared with me what had happened to her aunt and uncle in Las Vegas the past winter while I was in Colorado. It was an equally horrific story. I sent a text message to my dear friend Rosie, "God help me." Rosie called me within five minutes. I told her what was happening. She asked if I wanted to come over because she didn't want me at Hoyt's. I accepted her gracious offer. She came and picked me up after work, and I brought clothes for two days.

I went to bed at Rosie's, exhausted from the stress and strain, and slept fairly well. I woke up with a massive headache that relieved itself within minutes. I was beginning to see a glimmer of a game plan in the fog of my depression, and this was a good thing. Rosie gave me a huge hug that morning, happy that I'd accepted her offer for me to live with her and help her clean her house. She was such a sweet soul with a heart of gold. The amount of gratitude in my heart was overwhelming. It was like every hug was equivalent to winning the lottery. I cried tears of joy.

Two days later, I felt so much better. My head was clearing from the ammonia exposure. Her dogs are precious sweethearts, and there was love there. It was good to drink coffee on the back patio in the cool morning hour. After Rosie left for work, I watered the vegetable garden and the roses, giving them extra life force energy.

On Mother's Day in 2017, I was considering calling my mom and wishing her a happy Mother's Day. Was I strong enough? Would she throw venom at me? Who knew? Who cared anymore? I knew my mother was suffering. It had been four years. I really didn't want her suffering, as she had told me in her voice messages left on my phone. After visiting Rosie's mother's grave and her deceased husband's grave, I called my mom and wished her a happy Mother's Day. She was happy I called and said we used to have fun together. She thought it had been eight years since we spoke, even though it was only four. She told me my father was in a memory care unit in Phoenix.

The WhiteOne said they were waiting for me to do this. Now, my life would change again for the better. I truly hoped and had faith in this because I was tired of being without a foundation. I was truly grateful for all the support, love, and help I'd received so far. I was looking forward to the future, whatever it held for me. I was remaining positive and maintaining my vibration on a higher level than it had been the past week.

When I arrived back at Rosie's home from errands, I saw a leather sofa in the garage. I thought Rosie had really scored with that find because it was beautiful, and I loved the gold color. She said it wouldn't go in her house because of the color, but she wanted me to have it. It was a high-end leather sofa in very good shape. She said it would be a perfect sofa for an apartment. Positive messaging that I would be moving. Now I was getting excited about moving to an apartment by myself. Rosie converted her doll room into a bedroom for me. I was amazed at her generosity and feeling grateful. We are both very positive people and have the same outlook on life. Rosie was related to Hoyt, as they are both direct descendants of the famous American frontiersman, Kit Carson. We'd discovered this one day eating lunch at a restaurant when I had casually mentioned Hoyt's heritage.

I visited my dad on May 31. It was a lovely visit, and he asked about my business. He wanted to know if I had an office. We talked about Colorado and the Durango-Silverton train. We hugged and said "I love you" to each other. He remembered me and knew I was Barbara. I checked his very small room to make sure there wasn't anything that needed to be addressed and said hello to his roommate.

For several days, I debated in my mind between a single or two-bedroom apartment. Upon awakening the next morning, the answer came to me. Due to the increased traffic on the roads, the cost of gasoline, and maintenance on my vehicle, it made more sense to have a home office. I felt my dad had planted the seed in my mind when he asked me several times if I had an office. I can control the environment without much tasking. I knew God would send me the perfect clients, and they would be good people. This meant I would purchase a twin-sized bed mattress set and frame. The calming colors of sage green, lavender, and purple would be the design inspiration for the fabrics, and I began to see the room in my imagination. Everything begins with a thought and manifests accordingly. I believe this.

In June, I called Zeysan and spoke with him after having dreams of him for the past several nights. In last night's dream, he had a beautiful aroma about him, and it wasn't any cologne or soap. Recently, in his job rescuing children from sex trafficking, he'd sustained two bullets into his left shoulder. I wanted to know how he was healing. He said he was fine. I asked about my client's request for a spiritual qi gong class. Zeysan told me, "The disappointing news was the Shaolin in China have gone 'hierarchal,' meaning, there are no Shaolin monks teaching in California because it has turned into all about the money."

When Zeysan trained in the Shaolin temple in China, he was trained in martial arts fighting and the gentle monk healing aspect. Now, they were training monks to go out and do fighting to support the temples.

Basically, Shaolin had gone commercial. He did not know of anyone training in California, and the ones he knew had left that state.

"It really bothers me to give you this news. The next best thing would be for your client to obtain a Shaolin qi gong DVD and follow the instructions slowly," he said.

It was July 26, 2017, exactly one year since I'd held my Peter for the last time, and I thought of him that morning on the drive to my QHHT® client's home. I missed Peter. I had just become able to go to the restaurants and stores that we went to for years and not break down in tears. The only restaurant I couldn't go to was Olive Garden, the place of our first date after traffic school. I remembered he would go there for lunch while out and about in north Glendale. I just couldn't bring myself to go there yet. I knew to give myself time, and those feelings would pass.

On July 27, I went to the assisted living facility and visited my dad again. A woman named Peggy, who didn't talk, was sitting on the sofa with him. My dad wasn't engaging as much as last month. I asked him what he was watching on TV, and he said he didn't know. He didn't like being there. At 12:45 p.m., lunch was served. He was alone at the table because his roommate wasn't there. I sat with him in silence while he ate. I called Mom and told her where I was. She was happy I was doing this. It felt a great honor to sit with my dad and just be in a respectful mindset, remembering all he had done for me in his lifetime. It was a true honor to sit and be respectful to an elder. It felt so good to do this. I needed this. He was concerned I had nothing to eat, but I didn't mind. I told him I would eat when I went home. He didn't remember my mom visiting an hour earlier. When he finished eating, we walked over to the sofa. I gave him a hug and told him I loved him. He told me he loved me. When I told him I was leaving, he said, "I love you. Don't ever forget it."

It was like God was speaking to me. Source was telling me not to forget that I am loved. The ultimate separation—the original wound—remembered and healed in that moment. This was a gift. My heart chakra was wide open, and I was holding back the tears. My dad was a man of few words. When he spoke, he chose his words carefully from his career as a technical writer and speechwriter. I would always remember that moment for the rest of my life.

On August 1, 2017, I woke up during the night and received downloads of information for myself. The abrupt separation of my business and personal relationships with Virginia was necessary to show that I was moving into the New Earth, and she would stay on the Old Earth to continue her project. We had a celebration of this departure on the other side during our sleep. All was well! I loved receiving confirmation that we indeed were playing roles for each other. My work was evolving as I began to understand further and deeper into life projects that people engaged in.

In August, I interviewed Lance for an article about him and his service. I asked him about my recent painful left big toe. He added that I was releasing all the stuff I had processed about walking my path, trusting I would be provided for, and having faith that new clients were coming. I was moving forward in creating more books and a healing office for my clients where I could offer QHHT® and healing sessions and not have to drive long distances anymore. All this from my big toe!

That afternoon, Rosie asked me if I'd like to go to a second-hand furniture store. I had never been there, and I knew something was up. I checked inside of myself and received the green light, so I agreed to go. What happened next was astounding. I purchased a beautiful, lightweight wood end table that had a smaller lower shelf. Rosie spotted a Pfaff Performance 2056 sewing machine next to the used books for sale and suggested I go take a look at it. It had all the accessories. In fact, there were four of the same parts and a boatload of thread bobbins. The machine looked immaculate, with no scratches and no markings. I asked for someone to plug it in and see if it turned on. The top cover was not in its correct place, just laying on top, giving it the appearance of being broken. The presser foot lever would not move the presser foot. For thirty-nine dollars, I thought it would be a good idea to buy it and take it to the sewing store for an assessment. I checked in with the WhiteOne, who said, "This is why we wanted you to come to the second-hand store. This sewing machine is for you."

As I purchased the machine, Rosie gave me nineteen dollars in cash as a gift. While she moved her truck in the parking lot, I energetically cleaned the items with white light. A dust devil came as I stood outside with the machine. Then, I saw a heavy door with several locks on it blow open and then shut with a thundering sound. The message to me was a door of opportunity had opened. We went back to Rosie's home, and I cleaned the dust off the machine, plugged it in, and pressed the foot lever, pleasantly surprised that it worked.

A couple of weeks later, I received a report from the machine technician that the sewing machine was in pristine condition, inside and out. After he agreed to clean and oil the inside of the machine, I asked for my call to be transferred to the sales department. There I spoke with a sales lady and asked if I could have a sewing lesson for this machine. The original owner had left her registration form in the owner's manual, so the sales lady at the store gave me a free sewing lesson. She wasn't familiar with the machine either. It was not a new one, having been sold about eight to nine years ago at the same store. We learned the technology together. I loved my new machine and was grateful for it!! Several years ago, I'd placed a photo of a Pfaff sewing machine on my vision board for manifesting. Now the machine was in my reality, at the perfect price and the perfect time. I completed mending projects with this machine.

I found myself looking for a certified hypnotherapist training course in the Phoenix area, soon deciding on one that began the next month. When I spoke with the instructor, he said he'd just canceled the Phoenix course due to a lack of interest. He needed at least five people for the class. I was disappointed. It must have meant something greater or better was in store for me. I would continue to focus on my book and my work with people. I had the blessing that day of channeling healing for two clients. Dolores Cannon told me not to worry. Something wonderful would happen. She knew of my desire to acquire more skills and knowledge in hypnosis. I wanted to be able to offer more specific features in my business. I knew I would need the certified hypnotherapy credential if I was to incorporate my energy healing with hypnosis and advertise this down the road. Slowly, I worked toward acquiring the components for my hypnosis office and living on my own again in a two-bedroom apartment in Glendale, Arizona.

I was super focused on my book and had given myself a deadline

of the end of the year to have my manuscript ready for the first round
of editing. After the first round of editing, I would send it to Candace
for her to read and write the foreword for the book.

In the middle of October, my mother called and said she was not
feeling good and that there was nothing to live for anymore. She was
having suicidal ideation. I talked her out of it.

The next morning, I called her and went over to the house. We had
a conversation about her worries. She had an appointment with her
doctor and told me she'd been taking pain medication for the past four
years. She wanted to stop but felt awful if she didn't take it. She hadn't
slept well in four years while taking care of my dad. I called her again
two more times the next day, learning she was feeling better.

October 12, 2017, marked the one-year anniversary of Peter's ascension. I scheduled a deep tissue massage with Nicolette up in Wickenburg and drove up to her office. When we began the session, we
noted the neck area was much improved from last year, but my back
was a hot mess—knots of muscle fibers all over my back. My glu-
teus maximus muscles were extremely painful. My left hip was higher
than the right. I cried many tears. The pain from my muscles was felt
around my heart. My heart was feeling a great deal of sorrow. I just
didn't know what to do to release the issues. I repeated in my mind, "I
release, I release, I release."

October 18, 2017, my muscles were feeling better, and I went to
Deer Valley Park to do my tai chi. It felt good. My body felt out of
shape from sitting too much, writing, and rewriting the book. This was
one of the drawbacks of being an author. One must balance the stillness with the movement.

At the beginning of November, Rosie, Marge, and I went to Las
Vegas for a little fun while celebrating Rosie's birthday. Rosie and
Marge loved to gamble. They were so good at it, the hotel rooms were
comped. Marge stayed at Bally's, while Rosie and I roomed together
at the Wynn. Our room was beautiful, with a view of the Trump Hotel
and Casino. I brought my laptop with me so I could work on my *Time
Travels* book while enjoying the beautiful room.

Marge acquired free tickets to watch a paranormal hypnotist show
in the late afternoon at Bally's. While waiting in line, I said to Marge

that I didn't want to "go up on the stage, so don't try to coax me up there." Marge reciprocated the same sentiment, so we were in agreement. The show we attended was Frederic Da Silva's Mind Reading magic show. The way he selected participants was by throwing a stuffed elephant toy into the audience. The audience had to throw the toy three more times. When the elephant was thrown into the back, on the fourth pass, the woman who caught it said she didn't want to go up on stage, and she threw it high in the air toward the front. Where do you think it landed? That's right. In my lap! I said to myself, *This has Dolores Cannon written all over it!* How could I deny Dolores some fun? I stood up and walked on the stage.

Frederic had another woman on the stage, but not near me. We were given small whiteboards and a magic marker pen. I was asked to come up with a number from one to one hundred. I wrote the number down. The other woman had to guess what number I wrote and write it on her whiteboard. At the same moment, we turned our boards around to the audience. Both boards had the number 77 on them. The audience cheered. Life was good!

I felt like I was at a plateau in my life. I wanted to go forward and move into my new office, continuing the hypnosis work, the channeled healing work, write more books, and do some traveling. It was time to change my current situation. A good way to do that was through an intentional ceremony with a shaman. I called Lance, and we agreed to meet on October 30 at the same mountain we had years ago for a second shamanic opening ceremony.

CHAPTER 13

My Second Shamanic Opening Ceremony

I MET LANCE AT THE PHOENIX Mountain Preserve trailhead parking lot on a cloudy day. We hiked up the mountain and ended up on a peak higher than the one where we did the ceremony for my first shamanic opening in 2002. He found a spot with three partially buried rusty soda cans, one under a boulder. This was perfect.

He applied energy as I lovingly, slowly, and gently picked up the three cans. He emptied the dirt from the cans, and I placed them in a plastic bag to put in the garbage. Two of them had the name Shasta. As we did this ceremony, we saw a red-tailed hawk fly by and a black helicopter fly over the valley, but not near us. We created a sacred space. He placed five quartz crystals in a star pattern on the ground and asked me to state my intentions. I expressed that I wanted the whole enchilada about my work, my new relationship with a man who loves and supports me and who was awakened, my new office, abundant finances, a deeper and higher level of awareness, etc. He stood in the circle while I stood to the east and shook the rattle with my intention and focused on what I wanted to manifest and unfold. I moved into the circle and held the shaman staff. As I stared at Archangel Michael's image in the medallion inlaid into the wood of the staff, I stated my declarations. I channeled the mathematical star language, which transitioned into toning. When we finished, Lance sealed the ceremony as I stood behind him, shaking the rattle, then he instructed me to walk over to the promontory where the quartz striations were located and sit. There was an immense amount of energy there. I sat down and gave my gratitude to the mountain spirit, the angels, God, my Higher Self, Lance, and his Higher Self. I was given instruction from my guides to pick up a quartz rock for me. As soon as I said this to Lance, I saw a small—about an inch in diameter—quartz rock with four sides in a pyramid shape. He blessed it and charged it for me, and I placed it in my pocket.

We began the hike down the mountain, then stopped and waited. Lance saw a baby bat emerge out of its hiding place. As we approached closer, it flew away—such an auspicious totem for this ceremony. The bat tells us to face our fears and prepare for change. It was time to let go of what no longer suited me. Change and transformation are our blessings. The bat represented our ability to pierce barriers and be open to higher wisdom. It promises a new beginning of empowerment after we go through our transformation.

On the way down the mountain, I slipped and fell on my right buttocks, striking a pointed portion of a boulder. Sometimes, I need a kick in the butt from the universe to keep me on the path. This wasn't my favorite kind of messaging. We found the remains of a bird that had been eaten, and we each took a feather with a green edge to it. We then found a large white quartz rock that afforded us a seat to rest upon. As we were regenerating ourselves, Lance looked over and saw a large manmade hole in the ground, mostly covered by a Palo Verde tree. He looked up and saw that the hole was in direct alignment with the vein of quartz we could see along the mountain, where we'd held the ceremony, and specifically, where I'd sat after the ceremony.

Lance said, "Wow, that's where someone was digging for gold." A most auspicious metaphor about the inner work being done during this shamanic journey.

Lance called me the next day to see how I was. My neck had quit hurting. My buttocks and quads were a little sore, but I felt my strength gaining each day. I couldn't remember my dream from the night before but had received a download while in my bed last night. My body went into a full convulsive-type movement. I continued to focus on my book, my work, and my spiritual path.

At the beginning of November, while lying in bed reading Dr. Greer's book, *Unacknowledged, Part 1*, I read on pages eleven and twelve the story about the atomic bomb detonation on July 16, 1945, in Alamogordo, New Mexico. This was known as the Manhattan Project. I put the book down and received an energetic transmission. My body was shaking in a convulsive manner, and I was speaking the mathematical star language. Information was downloaded. I heard a voice within my mind say, *"This is why you were summoned to come to Earth. You are the one who has been dismantling the mechanisms that would cause nuclear destruction of planet Earth. You have special skills in this energy manipulation. This is why you saw yourself inside the Earth during the teleseminar you participated in. You destroyed the machines and devices that have been causing harm to others on the planet. Of course, there are others. You are not alone in your work. Please understand, dear one, this work was in a higher dimension to manifest in the third."*

This message confirmed for me that we are on planet Earth and performing tasks and jobs in other realms of existence. I didn't have the nuts and bolts of how this occurred and felt we are meant to focus on being human, explore our spirituality, and evolve in our consciousness. Part of that consciousness was knowing the bigger picture.

Then I was guided to look at the storage facility website where my belongings were located to see if a larger unit was available. I had been accumulating more furniture for my home office and apartment. They said they had two. I drove to the facility and paid for a corner unit right near the elevator. I felt so much better now that I had a bigger unit to store my stuff. I felt that I must stay in the Phoenix area, finish and publish my book, facilitate sessions, and conduct angel readings and channeled healings. In other words, I must be in service. I so much wanted a two-bedroom apartment where I was happy and had a hypnosis office. If God had something better or greater, then so be it.

In December, I had a dream where I walked outside and saw a rattlesnake around the corner of the yard. I tried to run but kept falling down, then managed to get the snake to go into the house. I was trying to yell, but it was hard to get the screaming words out. No one was helping me. No one was coming to my aid. The rattlesnake came out of the house, and I grabbed its neck so it wouldn't bite me. I was choking it to stop it from biting me. Its eyes were closed, but I was holding it and screaming. No one was coming to help me. I woke up sweating and upset. The snake was about change. The rattlesnake was about poison. The house was about my mind. Trying to scream words that wouldn't come out clearly was about speaking my truth. That no one was helping me was a message that I must depend on myself because I am strong and I am love.

I purchased a dream interpretation from Lance, where he explained to me that the snake in my dream was Peter. My guide told me to walk on the beach, and the snake would walk with me. Then I was told to sit down in the sand. The snake morphed into Peter. We got up and walked hand in hand away from the ocean and toward a dark cave. We walked into the darkness, and the cave turned into a jungle where we were both monkeys. He was my mate. I had a baby monkey. He went out exploring and didn't come back. He abandoned me. My heart was broken. I died of a broken heart. I went into the Light and met with my guides. We decided to do another lifetime together. This time, it was medieval times. Peter committed suicide because he couldn't be with me. We were of different social statuses. I was very distraught. Then, it was now this lifetime, and he abandoned me when he ascended. We walked out of the cave, and I gave him love. I sent him every aspect of myself. The snake was love.

On December 13, 2017, I felt different and at peace regarding Peter. I could now look at the entire eight years and see it from a different point of view. I saw it as the abandonment issue now resolving.

It was possible that my mother had had a change of heart. She called me on a Friday night and told me she acknowledged that I was the one who held the family together all those years. She asked me if she had ever thanked me for that. I told her no. I felt a little shocked as I attempted to comprehend and identify that this could be the changing of heart point. At the same time, I was feeling that I'd done my family a disservice by giving my power away so they didn't have to stand in their own power. She'd also changed her mind to not receive drugs anymore from the psychiatrist. She had chosen a psychologist to help her with her anxiety and panic attacks and was doing yoga once a week. This was a huge leap in her perspective.

The other night, I had a dream where George Clooney came into the lab with a sea anemone. The anemone morphed into a humanoid type of creature, and there was a cat with a hooded jacket helping it. The anemone creature reached back inside the jacket hood, scooped up some white goo substance, and placed it in the cat's eyes. The cat began to feel pain and started to die. I woke up upset.

George Clooney represented Peter because I associated George Clooney with a brand of coffee he endorsed in Switzerland when I was in Bern in 2010. Advertisements with George Clooney and the coffee were plastered everywhere in the city. A friend of Peter's referred to his coffee as "George Clooney coffee," and this image had stuck in my mind. The sea anemone represented spiritual diversity. The lab represented self-discovery. The cat represented independence. The jacket represented the exterior of what we show to the world or what we are trying to hide from the world. Hood and headwear signaled thought and attitudes we wanted to keep private or hidden. The white goo substance in the cat's eyes represented a lack of clarity, and the pain represented the thought of not being independent. My interpretation of the dream elements was that my Higher Self was telling me my independence from Peter would allow my spiritual walk to be revealed and presented to the world. I was the cat trying to help myself remain clear and independent in my self-discovery. The thought of being repressed through confusion and conformity meant I couldn't be my true and authentic self. This was against my mission and agreements, and it caused distress for me. My Higher Self was helping me to understand why Peter and I had to break the relationship in order for me to continue my spiritual walk.

Lance suggested I not think about there being any non-clarity of where I was. It was part of the process. I just had to view it like that. Anything that was not accepting of where I was could be a way of making it not clear. It added other energy into the mix. I was doing well, and I was where I was, and that's all there was to it.

I continued to facilitate QHHT® sessions for clients all over the Valley. Living with Rosie was so easy because we both have a love for sewing and making quilts. We made plans to attend the annual sewing and quilt show in January at the Veteran's Memorial Colosseum in Phoenix. I'd introduced her to making porcelain dolls back in

2003 when we'd worked together at the Hartford Insurance Company. I brought one of the dolls I had made to work to share one of my creations, and when she saw it, she inquired how I did it. I told her about the classes I'd attended each week, and the instructor who was considered one of the best in Arizona. I assured her that Judy Kitchen, the doll instructor at Sandy's Dream Dolls store, would not allow her to leave class without a beautifully painted and sculpted doll. I also told her all of the women who work at Sandy's Dream Dolls are experts in the field, including a woman named Patsy, who cowrote a book on porcelain doll competition judging, and Diana, who is a wealth of information and experience about dolls. This information inspired Rosie, so she came to the classes and made her own beautiful dolls.

It was January 2, 2018, when I celebrated Hoyt's birthday with him and our friend, Steve, at Mimi's Cafe for dinner. Hoyt was very upset with President Trump, thinking he was a crook. He didn't want to hear my perceptions. I didn't need to tell Hoyt my opinions because he was closed-minded. Even though I told him I read government documents, he said I didn't know what I was reading and I was stupid. I dropped into my heart and just allowed him to vent his anger, not holding onto it. I remained detached from the drama and the verbal attacks.

In the afternoon of January 11, 2018, I met Lance at the Phoenix Mountain Preserve entrance to perform a new healing meditation technique in a wash in the desert. We found a perfect place among the Sonoran Desert foliage of bushes and trees. We had a hummingbird with us. After Lance made the markings in the sand, I placed my crystal pointed upward at the correct spot, sat down cross-legged, closed my eyes, and placed my hands, palm up, on each knee. Lance held each hand between his, left one first, then the right. I channeled the healing language, and a Native American male energy chanted next. With a deep breath, it was done. When Lance held my right hand, more language and toning came forth from my vocal cords. I manipulated my star codes in my star field and removed a bunch of energy I no longer needed. It felt very powerful and balancing.

It was Lance's turn. As I watched him, while doing the same technique, his body was vibrating/shaking. I held sacred space with my palms facing toward him, arms down at my sides. I looked down and saw a quartz rock in the shape of a bat. When Lance began toning, I looked straight up into the clear blue sky and saw a jet flying right over us. A message came through that the benevolent extraterrestrials were watching us and agreed with our healing ceremony. Arcturians were with us.

For me, it was such a great honor to be in Lance's presence. It was like opening a Christmas gift. Lance was the gift. He had helped many people overcome their fears, prejudices, and negative beliefs that kept them stuck with illness and emotional pain. He was a conduit and a repository of love, compassion, wisdom, and knowledge. One would think that a man of this stature would be inaccessible. But no, not Lance. He was the embodiment of the divine, Jesus Christ—the Christ consciousness. I am blessed to call him my brother and my friend. When I referred a person to Lance, it was truly a gift for that person, and when their heart was open, they recognized this instantly.

On a morning in January 2018, while alone in the house, I did the Multi MerKaBa 5D meditation and added the sonic activation afterward. It was during the sonic activation that I saw a lotus flower opening slowly and gently in my mind's eye vision. The sensations felt new to me. I felt the eighth chakra much more intensely than the seventh chakra. I saw a group, the Kriya Yoga masters, standing around me, and I dialogued with Paramahamsa Hariharananda, confirming this meditation and breathing were in alignment with my Kriya Yoga.

On January 16, I woke up with my right eye red, swollen, and painful. I went hiking at Thunderbird Mountain in north Phoenix, and on the way back, I thought of Lance and the ceremony we did in the desert wash. I felt blessed to have received the gift of ceremony, knowing this was something that was appropriate for me. *Blessings to Lance*, I thought while looking over, and I had the impression that I was staring at a coiled rattlesnake. The rush of adrenalin went over my body and then dissipated when I saw there was no snake. I spoke with Lance that afternoon, and as soon as I started talking about this, I got the download. The toxin release was located in my eyes. I was going through a detox of the old programs, beliefs, and experiences of men not keeping their promises to me, betrayal in their behavior, and understanding this was something that was being released from me as well. I sent love to each of these souls. I sent love into myself, into my eyes, and into the situations I'd experienced. Clarity was coming into focus.

On February 23, I received a deep tissue massage minus 10-15 percent pressure to allow proper processing without residual pain like last month. I did the forgiveness technique regarding Peter. I was beginning to feel anger and allowing it to process in order to heal as much as I could, if not completely. The hidden anger must come forward to be released. We can't keep our emotions at arm's length or deep within us. So what was the anger about?

The anger was about leaving me, for leaving me abruptly, for walking out, for not allowing me to express what I was feeling because a new soul walked in, and it was not his fault or position to get the brunt of my anger. For cheating on me with a woman in Switzerland. For not communicating with me and letting me know that he was unhappy before announcing he was leaving. He gave me no choice and no opportunity to do something about it. For telling me to go find someone new. Why did he hug me goodbye the morning I left? Why did he leave his Skype conversation with his new girlfriend to hug me and say goodbye? Why did he "throw me out" of the ranch just like his father had he when he was eighteen, in the middle of winter in Switzerland, with just a jacket and fifty Swiss francs? Why?

I began processing more emotions the first weekend of March while sick with a head cold. Rosie had her family over for a reunion party, so I stayed in my bedroom with a sore throat and sinus drainage. I coughed all night. My mind was in la-la land. Rosie graciously let me have three doses of her cough medicine each night, and I was able to sleep and restore my health. I had to reschedule a QHHT® session until March 17 so I wouldn't have a nasal voice for the induction.

I received news from the hypnotherapy instructor. He would have a course in Phoenix starting in April. I was excited to enhance my hypnosis skills and learn more about hypnotherapy.

CHAPTER 14

Hypnotherapy Certification

I BEGAN THE BASIC HYPNOTHERAPY COURSE on April 10, 2018. We five students gave and received hypnosis sessions and techniques with each other. Mark Johnson, the instructor of Good Vibes Hypnosis, was a certified hypnosis trainer with the Michael Newton Institute. Both Mark and his wife, Lana, who was a psychic medium, were QHHT® practitioners. The course was taken over a four-day period. I appreciated Dolores Cannon's modality even more when I read the rationale behind hypnotic techniques. We learned that a person who was hypnotized would never do anything they wouldn't do, morally, ethically, or otherwise. In other words, if we didn't want to stand on our head, we wouldn't stand on our head. I was grateful for Mark and Lana taking their hypnosis training course on the road to other cities from their base in the Dallas area of Texas.

Driving in town, I began thinking of Peter and questioning if he really didn't walk out of his body. I knew this was my ego raising its head in doubt. I was trying to examine the truth of the situation, even though I already had evidence and confirmation. I had had conversations with my Higher Self while under hypnosis and while I was awake. Just when I was contemplating this, I looked over at the dental office across the street and saw the sign in the window that said, "Walk-ins welcomed." I did this automatically without searching. This is how the Higher Self gets us to see or find objects and messages. When you are walking in a parking lot, and you look down and see a coin, pick it up. It's a message from your Higher Self. It could be a message from a loved one who has crossed over. You don't know until you check inside of yourself.

My left upper outer thigh was painful, like a knife stabbing me when I laid on it at night. The pain was so intense it woke me up. I started a magnesium supplement that helped some. I also began walking on the treadmill in the house and using my two-pound weights for my upper arm conditioning and strength.

On Sunday, April 29, I received a shamanic healing with Lance for my left thigh pain. He discovered grief there and saw two glowing white extraterrestrial beings at the end of the table, next to my feet, during the session. This was an intense session. I definitely felt a release of old programs and thoughts.

At the end of May, I put my Expedition into the shop and was told she needed a lot of expensive work. AJ, at the car shop, asked me when I was planning on buying another vehicle. I replied, "Winter?" He just looked at me without expression. I added, "Summer?" He nodded his head yes. I knew right then and there that I had to go look for a car. I went to the Ford dealership where my friend's grandson worked and asked for him. He laughed when I said I wanted the monthly payments to be two to three hundred dollars. I said, "Okay, four hundred max." The national average for car loans at the time was $550 per month. I test drove a used Ford Explorer XLT 2015. It was nice, but the payments would be $520 per month. I left and went to my financial angel, Gloria, at my credit union. She gave me the information I needed to structure the car loan with the dealership because my credit history wasn't good enough for a car loan through them.

Within minutes of leaving the dealership, a 2013 Ford Edge SEL with just thirty-eight thousand miles came into the inventory, and my salesman called me. I told him I would come on Sunday to take a look at it. I drove to the dealership and test drove it. It was wonderful, and I really liked it. I spoke with AJ, and he checked the history. He had a good feeling about the Ford Edge too. My mechanic checked the vehicle's engine and gave me the thumbs up. I bought the Ford Edge and named her Crystal because she's white and has crystals in the paint that sparkle in the sun. I made plans to refinance the loan to a lower premium the following year and reduce my payments by half for the rest of the loan term.

On May 13, 2018, I completed the advanced hypnotherapy course with Mark and Lana. In this course, we learned that hypnosis could be done during surgery. I watched a video of a woman having her thyroid gland removed without anesthesia. There was no bleeding, and she was awake the whole time in a hypnotic state. We learned and practiced parts therapy, which helped a person heal their inner trauma memories.

I drove to Wickenburg on the twenty-second for a massage with Nicolette. We examined my left hip, which was extremely painful to the touch, and my entire back was filled with knots. I purchased magnesium oil spray, added turmeric and water to my diet, practiced meditation, and used my stress reduction techniques. I did more releasing of Peter and told him I couldn't make myself sick over the grief anymore because I had a lot of work and living to do. Nicolette recommended I go to a chiropractor.

I remembered reading about Dr. Shawn Warwick, a chiropractor who did energy work, on Ann Albers's referral list on her website and scheduled a session with him. My first session was one and a half hours of energy work. He also adjusted my spine in a very gentle manner.

I returned to Dr. Warwick in one week because my hip was hurting more, and I was limping. The pain was waking me up at night. I thought it would be just a few minutes, but I was in a large room with four other people for over two hours. My body shook at one point. Then he removed something from my left ear area. I saw red on the left side of my vision and orange on the right side. Then he came over and did more energy work. I began speaking the mathematical star language, and it went into a scream, much like an exorcism. I smelled burning sage afterward.

The next day, I received a two-hour deep tissue massage with Nicolette, then returned to Dr. Warwick on my scheduled two-week checkup. This time, I was placed in a private room. After several energy adjustments, I could feel Dr. Warwick still in the room working on me. It made me laugh because this was what happened for my energy work clients. I noted Dr. Warwick used the same words and the same phrases when he talked with me.

By July 1, 2018, my left hip was better. At least I could sleep through the night without intense pain and do my tai chi and qi gong, though yoga was still painful. I just couldn't do it. I spoke with Zeysan about this, and he said it was because I was healthy. The tai chi he'd taught us helped all the organs to vibrate at their healthy frequency. Yoga tried to make all the organs vibrate at the same frequency, and this causes discomfort in the body.

By July 3, my left hip was feeling 90 percent better. I received my first book cover version from the artist for my *Time Travels* book, and I think the artist nailed it. On July 20, 2018, the left hip pain was gone, but I had pain in the left thigh. It had moved down my leg.

I asked my Higher Self when and where I would be moving into my own place. The response I heard was, "Complete your course, and you'll be tickled pink with where you will be moving. This is all we will say at this time." This information was good enough for me because I trusted them and myself.

On July 13, I sent my homework assignment to Mark and then waited for my hypnotherapy certification.

In the early morning of July 22nd, I woke up sick to my stomach. I had three loose stools, then vomited three times into my trash basket. The room was spinning, and I felt very weak. I tried drinking water but kept throwing it up. I spent the day in my room, taking sips of water only. I couldn't tell if it was food poisoning or gastroenteritis. Time would tell. I didn't feel I had a fever. The next day, I felt weak and started myself on full liquids, then I was able to eat a piece of toast and yogurt. I was thankfully able to progress to my Rainier cherries, as I didn't want to waste this wonderful fruit.

Two days later, I had to move two clients to other days in the schedule because I was still weak, pasty looking, and slightly dizzy that morning. I needed to take it easy a bit longer. I was still alive, loving my work, writing more books, and thankful for it. I looked forward to moving to my new nest, feeling much better on the twenty-sixth.

On July 31, I drove up to Wickenburg for my monthly deep tissue massage with Nicolette. The drive was easy and took exactly one hour. The night before, my left thigh had ached with pain deep near the bone. It didn't matter which way I positioned my body because my thigh was on fire. Nicolette found a muscle spasm in the thigh. We decided the TENS (transcutaneous electrical nerve stimulation) unit and massage of the muscle before going to bed may help. I purchased a TENS unit at the local pharmacy.

After the massage, I drove to the spot Peter and I used to go to look at the Sombrero Ranch from across the wash. I gazed upon the home where I'd spent eight years of my life with him and didn't cry. I felt peace, gratitude, and love. I then imagined the portal above the house and sent everyone love. I felt a sense of more closure to the processing of this blow to the heart. If I was to assist in the ascension, then I must move forward in love and gratitude. No more sorrow. No more sadness.

On July 31, 2018, I participated in Gma's Canadian Rockies portal grid formation teleseminar. Gma and I were dolphins playing in the water at Lake Louise. After we completed the job, we lifted out of the lake, straight up to the stars, and met Archangel Michael. He placed his sword on my left shoulder and poured love into my heart. Gma and I went into our whale forms in the Pacific Ocean. My physical feet were very warm during the meditation. The music was a seamless play of melodies. I didn't notice any music changes as others did.

I returned my focus to working on my QHHT® session stories book, *Time Travels*.

CHAPTER 15

Time Travels:
Exploration of Lives Remembered

O N AUGUST 6, 2018, FORMATTING experts began working on the manuscript. The project coordinator, Rafael, wrote in his email message that the book cover would be completed, including the back cover copy, in a couple of weeks or so. I was very excited this book was finally coming into reality. Last November, Lisa Montgomery had given me the most auspicious day to publish this book. On October 8, 2018, *Time Travels: Exploration of Lives Remembered* would be published.

I received my very first acupuncture treatment for my left thigh pain from acupuncturist Julie Rae. She was most gracious, gentle, caring, and thorough in her history taking. The treatment room and her home had good energy. Julie shared with me that her birthday was the same date Dolores passed over. I filled out the history form and then changed into my shorts while she went to her office to prepare the treatment plan. Julie said I was the epitome of health. She said my tongue was healthy with the white coating and something about the veins looking good. When she honed in on the left thigh with the scar, I shared the story about the ET implant removal. Julie said that the pain I was experiencing could be from this too. I had not thought of that before. Certainly, cellular memory could be a valid reason. I laid down on the treatment table. After explaining what could be expected, she began inserting the needles. There was a little discomfort in the right-hand needles, but not intolerable. Everything settled down quite nicely. She gave me a remote ringer bell in my left hand in case I needed to summon her, then dimmed the lights and placed Japanese flute music on at the perfect volume. She left the room and returned in ten minutes to check on me.

I was at total peace. My Higher Self showed me a padlock with the lock opening. *Nice visual, WhiteOne!* I thought. A picture was worth a thousand words, and the information came in easily. This acupuncture session felt more like a day at the spa. Very relaxing. I could feel the energy moving in my body.

Almost two weeks later, when my left thigh was hurting that night, I placed the TENS unit on for a fifteen-minute massage. This helped greatly, and I was able to return to sleep.

I received an intuitive feeling that if I was to have a place to live, it might be a good idea to start looking at apartments. I searched on the internet and found six complexes to check out. I visited two a day over a six-day period, then sat down and narrowed the selection to three, then two complexes. One of my criteria was to have a window over the kitchen sink. Another was for an upper-level two-bedroom apartment for a home office. I applied online to the apartment complex I'd moved to back in 2005, when I'd left Hoyt, then left it up to God. I was approved in less than one hour. I was tickled pink! WhiteOne was right again.

On August 22, in my second acupuncture session, Julie did "fire with cupping," which was very interesting. With my eyes closed, I jokingly asked, "What are you going to do? Put me on fire?" I opened my eyes and saw Julie with a tall flame in the air. Yikes! I slipped into trust mode and watched the master at work. She placed the fire into the round glass cup, then withdrew the cup and placed it immediately on my left thigh, rubbing it around on the skin. She did this several times, and it didn't hurt at all. She explained the cupping helped draw the stagnant energy deep inside to the surface. Julie finished the treatment with a vibrating massager over the hip and leg area.

On August 31, in my third acupuncture session, Julie used the needles and finished with the fire cupping. My last acupuncture session was on September 7. I had no pain and was very pleased with the results. Julie said that I was done and did not need to return.

On September 28, 2018, I drove up to Sedona, Arizona, and had lunch at the Mariposa Latin Inspired Grill. This butterfly-themed restaurant was one of the five food establishments in Sedona owned by executive chef Lisa Dahl. I chose to sit on the outdoor patio with the magnificent views of the red rocks and flowers. I had the vegetarian filet with grilled portobello mushrooms, caramelized onions, and chipotle on a bun, along with a side of three seed cilantro slaw and a key lime tart with whipped cream, fuchsia flowers, and berries for dessert. It was heavenly. I met a lovely couple from New York City sitting next to me. The wife was a psychic medium and said she could see my red aura, which extended out far from my body. I didn't mention to her that I was on my way to Prescott Valley for my aura photo session with Reverend Liz Johnson, who does Kirlian photography. I shared with the couple some activities they could do in the Sedona area since they were staying there for four days. This goes to show us that you never know who you will meet along the way in your life and what delightful surprises the universe has in store for you.

In the mid-1990s, I had an aura photograph taken of me in an angel shop in Sedona. I've since lost that photo. I do remember a magenta color above my head, and gold and white colors surrounded me. When that photo was taken, I remember I'd placed my right hand on a metal plate.

Kirlian photography was invented in 1939 by Semyon Kirlian, and it is a photographic process that reveals visible auras around objects in photographs by applying a voltage of current to a metal plate. An object to be photographed is placed on the film, and an electrical coronal discharge between the object and the metal plate occurs that is caught on film. People did not know about the Kirlian photography phenomenon until the 1970s.

We now have computers using biofeedback technology to produce an electronic image of a person's aura. We have energy pathways in our bodies called meridians. Impulses traveling through the meridians are converted to an electrical frequency, displayed as colors and patterns in a person's aura. The colors are expressed qualities and traits unique to the person being photographed.

Recently, a friend of mine suggested I have my aura photo taken in Sedona. The same week I planned to do so, the great trance channel of Dr. Peebles, Summer Bacon, posted an article about her aura photo taken of herself and of her channeling Dr. Peebles, who had been a civil war surgeon, spiritualist, author, naturopathic physician, and world traveler. When he died in 1922 at the age of 99.9 years old, he was channeled by a close friend four days later. Since then, others have channeled him. He has a very distinct Scottish accent. In my opinion, Summer was the greatest trance channel I'd ever witnessed. She taught me how to channel. The aura photographer who provided the service was Liz Johnson[29] of Prescott, Arizona, a close friend of Summer.

My curiosity peaked, and I wondered if I could do the same with my Higher Self. I called Liz and made an appointment. After a short visit and lunch in Sedona, I drove over to Prescott for my photo session. The photography was fast and easy. I sat down and placed each hand on metal plates. There was absolutely no electrical sensation. It was like placing your hands on a countertop in the kitchen. About a minute later, I channeled the mathematical star language that plays in my mind 24/7, speaking it out loud for about ten seconds. The WhiteOne announced their presence and spoke directly to Liz in the English language. The photo was taken while I was in a trance.

The photographic process was easy and fast, and Liz was spot on during the aura reading. She said, "The energy on your right side is the energy you put out to the world. This is how people sense you. Very passionate. Very creative. You have a very strong conviction about the things you believe in. Things you hold dear to your heart. And you'll fight to the death to stand up for what you believe in. It's a good thing. You have a wonderful command of language. You're good at articulating and expressing yourself. You are kind of like the life of the party. You have a great sense of humor. People are drawn to you. Have you noticed when you're out, people want to stand next to you? It's because you have this wonderful energy. You make them feel good just standing next to you. You are very much a free spirit. You like to march

---

29   http://auraliz.com/index.html

to the beat of your own drum. (I had spoken those words earlier that morning with a slightly different twist: 'I step to the beat of a different drummer.') You don't like people telling you how to do stuff. Above your head (referring to the color in the photo) is where you are right now. You are in a creative cycle right now, but you're putting a lot of thought into it. You're not just jumping in willy-nilly. You're thinking about and putting a process into what you want to create next—really good energy. Your aura is huge, by the way. Your aura is probably four to five feet out.

"You have this beautiful green orb over your heart chakra. It tells me two things. You truly speak all of your truth through your heart, and you've been working on something in your heart. You have done a lot of work on this because the color is not very deep. You're doing good. (Liz was spot on about my heart chakra because of the personal processing I had been going through for the past two years about Peter and the blow to the heart experience. I was at the tail end of it.) Beautiful photograph. I love that we can hardly see you in there!"

On October 2, 2018, I had a dream where my right hand was bitten by a black widow spider, and the whole hand turned black. Then someone said to pour hydrogen peroxide on it. I did, and the hand returned to normal. Then I was changing a baby diaper. The baby was happy, and it brought me joy to see the happy baby. From Mary Summer Rain's dream dictionary, black widow spider meant an extremely dangerous individual or relationship in one's life. There was an individual who threatened me, but my Higher Self had removed the threat after I requested they take care of the situation. This dream was confirmation that my request had been heard and acted upon, as confirmed by the hydrogen peroxide component. Hydrogen peroxide was a purification conduit for healing. The baby diaper was about the false innocence of my effort to control the situation. I knew I had to give it up to the universe because I was not qualified to deal with that particular situation.

On October 4, 2018, I noted it had been a month since my last acupuncture session, and the left thigh and hip were perfect. No discomfort whatsoever. However, an old ailment showed up. The right greater toe had dislocated, and the pain was excruciating. I was unable to bend my foot in a normal fashion and hobbled when walking. I returned to

Julie on October 3 for an acupuncture session for this toe. She placed the needles in my left hand, left thumb, left foot, right leg. I also had a mild spasm of the plantar tendon.

On October 18, 2018, *Time Travels: Exploration of Lives Remembered* was published. It felt so good to click on that "publish" button. I moved into my apartment on October 19, 2018. A dear friend and her sixteen-year-old daughter helped me move the items from the storage unit into the apartment. It was perfect timing to leave Rosie's home because her adult son was on his way to live with her again. Two days later, I began unpacking. I unpacked boxes for the remainder of the week. My body screamed in pain each night from all the movement. Epsom and sea salt baths helped greatly. My large toe didn't give me any dislocation problems whatsoever.

On October 23, I went to Dr. Warwick for an energy treatment for my big toe and a general tune-up due to my muscles hurting. At one point, I passed out from the brain rewiring he did. And this was good. While driving back home from Dr. Warwick's and stopped in traffic, I was rear-ended on the Loop 101 freeway. The message from my Higher Self was to slow down even more. My lower back was sore since it was a low-impact collision. The next day, I decided to change my perspective and pretend the other driver and I were playing bumper cars. At that moment, I received instantaneous healing. The discomfort went away immediately.

On December 23, I was interviewed by Candace Craw-Goldman on her show, *Quantum Healing with Candace*, through *InD5 Radio*, hosted by Gregg Prescott. This was done live on Facebook with the Zoom video platform. I felt it went well. My website virtual assistant, Rose, uploaded the video to my website so people could learn about QHHT® sessions and how I facilitated them.

December 30, 2018, I held my *Time Travels* book in my hand. Staring at Dolores's book on my bookcase library, I asked her if she would help get more people to write reviews on my book's online listing. I heard her clearly reply, *"What do you think I am doing here, twiddling my thumbs?"* Her response shocked me, and at the same time, it made me laugh. I called Candace and told her what happened. Candace said,

"Oh, that's exactly what Dolores would say!" I was understanding more that I had a 24/7 connection with the master.

On December 31, as I do every year, I spent the evening by myself in my apartment, meditating and sending the world peace and love. I was feeling grateful for my family, especially my parents.

CHAPTER 16

My Dad's Passing

O N JANUARY 6, 2019, I prepared for my MerKaBa program renewal. As I was going through the programs and setting up the verbiage, the WhiteOne came through, strongly advising me not to take down the old programs. I had received upgrades in my light codes, and it was no longer necessary to take them down. They had given me special enhancements. However, they did say if I wanted to recite the protection list of substances and technology that are not conducive to human beings, plus add the new ones, it would be okay. They said it was because I had evolved in my fifth-dimensional expression and that all was being taken care of. I was in the energetic flow of manifestation for prosperity, health, and grace. The physical evidence was showing up in my reality and consciousness.

My mother was either sleep-deprived, or the dementia was setting in fast. This could have been a combination of the two. She was making no sense on the phone and in a constant meltdown whenever I called to say hello. I knew she was helping me remain calm and centered. Mom was releasing big time. I prayed for her and sent her love, comfort, peace, and rest. This seemed to be working quite nicely, to have healthy boundaries as everyone should have.

On January 18, 2019, I had a dream where I saw a large, tall, white building with a sign that read, "Switzerland." There were other names, but I didn't remember them. I said, "Oh, look, there's a store for Switzerland. I've got to go check that out." I went into the store and saw a lot of people working, making watches and jewelry. There were many Swiss items for sale, including food. I looked up and saw the Rado watch sign. It looked like a TV screen shape. I wanted to go to the elevator and had a hard time finding it. I walked around until I saw it behind the front welcome desk. As I walked back there, there were multiple elevators, but they moved sideways, not up and down. One had a brass sign with an arrow pointing to the right that said, "Amethyst." Another one had the arrow pointing to the left and said, "Rose Quartz." Swiss stands for finances and banking. A watch and clocks stand for the quote, "It's now time." Elevators moving sideways stand for focusing on strength into the masculine. Rose quartz was focusing on love into the feminine.

Shaman Lance concurred this was an auspicious dream, meaning I had attained an accomplishment.

My apartment refrigerator had recently been replaced because of the noise it was making. The new one was completely quiet. Refrigerator means "chill out." Be calm. This was what was meant by expanding our awareness—noticing what was occurring in our physical reality and applying the meaning and message to our inner beingness.

On January 22, 2019, I received a deep tissue massage from Nicolette. I no longer cried about Peter and was more at peace, ready to write about the blow to the heart and share the inspiration and strength I had gathered. It was time to start putting the Expansion book together for publication. I was experiencing that when we simplify our life, we notice everything is provided for. This is because we need less, and as a result, the money goes farther, and there's no clutter or overwhelming feeling. When someone gives us an object, we can really feel the prosperity because there are not a lot of other objects in our living environment that dilutes the sensation of the new object.

While purchasing a vintage dining room table and chairs, a woman in a Mini Cooper backed into the front of my vehicle. No one was inside my vehicle, and three of us yelled for her to stop. It didn't work. I kept calm and told the woman this was a case for her insurance company to handle. No one was seriously injured. We exchanged information and parted ways.

On January 30, after receiving a rental car to use while my car was being repaired, I drove home and prepared to go hiking. With my hands full of hiking boots in a box, a walking stick, a water bottle, two sets of keys, and my belly pack, I received a premonition halfway down the twenty concrete stairs that I would fall. With the next step down, I fell. I knew to go with the fall and relax into it. I flipped over and cracked my right leg on the steps. I landed on the next to last step, sitting up and a little dazed. A guy walking by asked if I was okay. I told him, "I think so." I felt pain in my right shin, pulled up my yoga pants, and saw the bloody cuts from my kneecap down to the ankle. I gathered the spilled items on the ground and limped up the stairs, then home to lay down on my sofa with an ice pack on my leg. I went to sleep, knowing it was important for me to be out of my body so my Higher Self physicians and beings could work on the muscles and tissues. I was sore for the next three days as though someone had beat me up. I later discovered my inner right ankle was bruised, but there were no broken bones. I called Julie and asked about an acupuncture session for tissue trauma, and we scheduled the session.

On Saturday, the 2nd of February, I attended an online hypnotherapy conference. In the evening, I drove to Scottsdale and participated in the Feng Shui Arizona Chinese New Year ceremony and celebration. Everyone was kind, supportive, and in a good mood. I put new business cards in my books that Lisa had for sale in her store.

For the past two weeks, my dad had been in a behavioral health facility for evaluation of behavior problems. He had punched a caregiver in the face and broken her nose. My dad didn't normally hit people. In my entire life, I had never seen nor heard of him hitting someone other than us children for disciplinary reasons. Two days later, he was found unresponsive on the floor. He was taken to the emergency room and diagnosed with two pulmonary emboli (blood clots) and a mass in his lung. It was possible my dad's oxygen saturation had decreased to a level where the brain malfunctioned, and his cognitive ability was impaired for normal processing of information. This could have made him belligerent and caused him to lash out, striking the caregiver in the memory care unit. I wasn't informed of this episode until Monday, the 4th of February. Laying in the telemetry unit of the hospital, he was sleeping when I entered his room. I observed him and made my assessment, scanning the room and making note of the equipment and his vital signs. His cardiac monitor showed atrial fibrillation. An atrial fibrillation rhythm is the quivering electrical conduction of the upper chambers of the heart, which causes erratic contractions, thus allowing for stagnation of the blood in the upper chamber. This is a known cause of blood clot formation, strokes, and heart failure. Atrial fibrillation causes a 25 percent reduction in cardiac output, thus reducing the amount of oxygen traveling to the organs and tissues in the body. People feel a decrease in their energy level because of this blood flow reduction. My dad's nurse came into the room, making notes in the computer system at his bedside. I inquired about his status and the plans for his hospitalization. With our talking, my dad woke up and recognized me. A few minutes later, my mom arrived, and we visited with my dad together. He kept asking, "What is that?" He pointed to the speaker cover on the ceiling. It was as if he'd turned into an inquisitive child, unfamiliar with the components of a typical hospital room with ventilation duct covers, speaker covers, a sprinkler system apparatus, and so forth. His pulmonologist came to visit and evaluated his respiratory status. The doctor said he would monitor my dad's progress, as there was a mass found on the chest X-ray. Seeing my dad was comfortable after his meal, my mom and I left the hospital.

A week later, on the 25th of February, I received a text message from my brother that my dad was in the emergency room. I drove south of where I lived and found my dad in a ninety-five-bed emergency department of a hospital where I had once worked. He was resting after eating a full meal, having been very hungry when he regained consciousness. After a couple of days, he was transferred back to the behavioral health facility. My brother walked into my dad's room and found him crying. He was in a locked unit with paper clothes, no television, no books, and nothing but the walls to stare at. We found out they weren't feeding him, and he was a diabetic. The staff gave my dad his diabetic medicine but no food. My brother spoke with the case manager and facilitated an expedited transfer to a higher level of care at the assisted living facility. My dad was moved immediately.

I visited my dad several times. On March 17, he was lying in bed, extremely sedated. I showed him his birthday card and hung it on the bulletin board in the room. I sat down next to him and talked. He couldn't respond with intelligible words. He'd lost twenty pounds and was very sedated by the Haldol tranquilizer medication to keep him from being violent. While he slept, I placed my right hand on his heart. I told him telepathically that it was okay for him to leave this earthly existence. We wanted him to be happy and at peace.

I recalled his life story.

My dad was born in 1931on St. Patrick's Day in Mayfield, New York. He was the first of two sons. He played the trumpet in the high school orchestra and was a member of the thespians. According to the notes his teachers wrote to my grandmother, he was smart and a good student. Upon graduation from high school, my dad worked at General Electric in Schenectady, New York. He found rides with coworkers for the thirty-two-mile commute. His father, my grandfather, Jerome Becker, worked in the metal fabrication factory of General Electric in Schenectady. My dad met my mother at a cousin's wedding. My mother was the maid of honor, and my dad was a groomsman. My dad wrote down my mother's car license plate number so he could track her down. My youngest sister found that piece of paper before the estate sale of my parent's home. My parents began dating, then married in 1951. My dad had to ask for permission from his parents to marry my twenty-one-year-old mother because he was only nineteen years old, a statutory minor in New York. The legal age of an adult back then was twenty-one.

They were married in the Catholic Church, and the reception was held in the basement of my mom's sister's house. People entertained in their basements in Upstate New York back then. After a January wedding and a honeymoon to Niagara Falls, NY, my parents lived with my dad's parents until they saved up their money to purchase a home at 31 James Street in Gloversville, NY. My mom worked at Nathan Littauer Hospital in Amsterdam, where she received her diploma for nurse's training to become a registered nurse.

My mom became pregnant with my oldest brother, giving birth to him that same December of their first year. The home they bought had an apartment upstairs. My parents lived in the lower part of the home and rented the upper half. This didn't work out so well because my mom worked nights, and the children upstairs would play their musical instruments during the day. They had to ask the renters to leave. My mom worked sporadically and had to care for my brother. A year later, she gave birth to my second oldest brother. Instead of having daycare for my brothers, my mom stayed home. Two years later, I was born in 1955. My parents could not afford the mortgage, so they sold the house and moved into my dad's parent's home again. They lived there from September to the following March. My grandmother was difficult to live with, and my mom needed to have her own nest to raise her children. Most people would tell you not to live with your in-laws; however, there are circumstances where nothing else is viable. Each generation must be allowed to raise their children in their own way.

My dad went to night school and received further training in electronics. He acquired a position with General Electric in Syracuse, New York. My parents moved us to Camillus, a suburb of Syracuse, in 1958. We lived at 113 Barclay Road. My mom worked nights and slept during the day. I remembered a day when I was three years old, and my mother was asleep in the living room recliner. I crawled up on the kitchen counter and stood up to reach the top shelf of the cabinet where the baby aspirin was kept. I opened the bottle (back in the fifties, they had not invented childproof containers for medicine), took out one orange-flavored aspirin, and ate it. To me, it was candy. I put the lid back on and replaced the bottle in the cabinet, never telling her this story until 2020. This was the only time as a child that I took medicine without my parents' knowledge. I imagined my Higher Self wiped out any desire for me to repeat this dangerous behavior! For this, I was grateful.

Living in Camillus, our neighborhood consisted of one long, curved street. There were plenty of children to play with back then. Our house had a breezeway connecting the detached garage, and we had a swing in our backyard to play on. Around the perimeter of the house, my mother grew bearded irises of many colors and pink roses. She would cut bunches of irises for me and wrap them in a wet paper towel, wax paper, and aluminum foil for me to take to my first- and second-grade schoolteachers. There was a baseball diamond behind the house for the boys to play. We climbed up an apple tree, where a tree fort was made of wood boards. My mom gave us children and our friends pots, pans, and steel bowls to gather wild raspberries and blackberries from the edge of the forest behind our house. We flew kites in the spring. Our milk was delivered in glass bottles by a milkman and left on our breezeway by the kitchen door. I remembered the goat's milk that came in root beer-colored bottles. Life was good.

In the winter, my siblings and I made snow angels and snow tunnels outdoors. We had sleds and round metal saucers with handles to slide down the hill behind and between our house and my best friend's house next door. Someone had a long toboggan for us children to ride down the hill and out to the street. I sucked on icicles and slipped on icy sidewalks. Mom served us hot cocoa when we came in from playing all day in our snowsuits. My favorite time of the winter day was at dusk, just before going into the house for dinner. I remembered standing in the snow on the front lawn, listening and appreciating the peaceful silence of the world, gazing upon the blue-violet sky. Snow absorbs sound, and that was why the environment was quieter.[30] Life was beautiful.

My dad was transferred to Daytona Beach, Florida, to work on the Apollo Space Program. NASA hired ten thousand computer technicians to work on the Saturn rocket for the manned space mission to Earth's moon and back. Specifically, my father wrote logistic equations for the computers to detonate the explosives on the space capsule upon splashdown into the Atlantic Ocean, opening the windows for the astronauts to egress into the water. Those windows were welded shut for space travel. I imagined that the astronauts could not have one iota of claustrophobia in their work! I was still in awe of the men and women who dared to venture beyond our Earth's atmosphere. My dad also wrote and edited technical manuals for General Electric. We left New York in the winter of 1963.

In Florida, my dad was a Boy Scout leader, and my two brothers were members of the local troop. For a short while, my mother was a Brownie troop leader. My girl scout leader never took the first aid course required for our troop to go camping, so I was jealous of my brothers being able to go camping and to the Boy Scout Jamboree

---

30   https://bit.ly/3shEQPU

each year. To make up for this lack of activity, my friend Dianne and I camped out in her backyard. Those were fun times when we would stay up late at night, play games, and watch scary movies on the television.

On February 13, I spent the night at my mother's home to give her a reason to have a good night's sleep. It worked, and we awoke in the morning and went to Mimi's Cafe for breakfast. We ate half the food we were given and brought the rest home.

My hair spoke with me and said it wanted to grow longer. I went over to Supercuts hair salon and had Kelsey cut my hair. I felt younger and more vibrant without the hair hanging down on one side of my face.

What was interesting was my mother's questions. "Why are you visiting so much? Am I going?"

I asked her, "What do you mean?"

She replied, "That I am going to die."

I told her I was visiting because it was nice to have someone in the house and spend the night and visit.

She responded, "Oh yes!" As I left, she said, "You are a caring person."

I sat in meditation and noticed that there was no separation between anything or anyone. That everyone was me. All the furniture, walls, and objects were me, God, and the Oneness. I realized that everything and everyone, including the entire universe, was a thought of God. I love God. I could see once again that all was in right order, and I could be at peace. I spoke with Zeysan later that day about embracing our evil as well as our good because we were capable of both. This is the totality of us. This is where choice comes into play. We choose to be good or bad. We choose to do good or do bad. It's up to us.

On March 8, I had a dream where I saw extraterrestrial vehicles take off and become clouds. Then I saw these vehicles flying transdimensionally into a building, without harm to the building or the craft. I explained to others how this worked. I really enjoyed this dream.

On March 19, 2019, I meditated using the Angel Treasure hill/cave meditation. AngelTreasure, my guide, came down on his painted horse. It had been a while since I'd done this meditation—years. He asked me to walk with him into the darkened cave. As we walked on the cool green grass, I stopped and cried. I told him I missed Peter. He held me and said, "I know." I told him, "I'm sorry. It's just taking longer than I thought." AngelTreasure said, "It's okay." We walked into the cave, and I saw a fire on the ground, deep inside. I sat down. There was nothing and no one to talk with or confront. I fell asleep. I woke up at 2:22 p.m. AngelTreasure said, "Congratulations, you've mastered your fear. You came into the cave without hesitation or question. You trusted yourself, and you trusted me, your guide." We walked out through another path, and I found myself walking on the wet sand of the beach. Leo, my lion totem, was running toward me, kicking up his heels. We gave each other a high five and hugged.

I was at Home Depot buying a can of paint when I looked at my phone and saw my mom had called and left a message that my dad was passing. I called her and told her I was on my way. I drove to the facility, briefly signed in, and walked up the stairs and to the room where my mom was sitting next to my dad. My siblings and their spouses and children were there. I walked straight into the room, squatted down, and placed my right hand on my dad's chest to make sure he had left the body and was not suffering in any way outside the body. He was in the room, looking at us, though I could not share this with my family because I didn't want to cause any fear or concern.

My dad had died at 12:52 p.m. on the 20th of March in 2019 before I arrived at the assisted living facility. He had been given several doses of a tranquilizer and antianxiety medication during the death process, according to his nurse. The male nurse told me his legs became mottled. Cheyne-Stokes breathing followed. The nurse gave him a Tylenol suppository for pain. The hospice nurse was called. The chaplain was summoned. And then my dad had stopped breathing. I wished the nursing staff had called us sooner. I wanted to be there at his side.

After the ambulance attendants took my dad's body to the funeral home, we went over to my parents' home. My brother started talking about a funeral, and I suggested that instead of spending all that money, we could have a celebration of life lunch at P.F. Chang's. This would allow more money to be left for Mom. Others agreed, so we quickly made plans for Saturday to give my sister Maureen and her family time to fly in from California. We could only invite twenty people for the private dining room, and my brother, Don, took care of calling everyone.

On the drive back to my apartment to pick up my travel bag so I could spend the night with my mom and finish drying my clothes in the dryer, I saw a license plate: AZDO315. I interpreted the plate like this:

Archangel Azrael, the angel of hospice, ministers, and mediums who help people.

D: Dad.

O: He's telling me he made it "over."

31: Dad was born in 1931.

5: Change.

March 21 was my birthday, one day after my dad's passing. At 3:33 a.m., I woke up to the sound of a freight train. My dad loved trains. I felt my dad taking advantage of the spiritual hour when it's easier for messages to come through. I also felt he was telling me happy birthday.

On the 22nd of March, I took Mom to the Heritage Funeral Home to submit a nice photo of my dad for the bookmarks to be made as a memento. Before we left the driveway, a red-tailed hawk flew over and circled the house. I knew that was my dad. We stopped for a moment and watched the bird, then drove to the cemetery in El Mirage so we could see where the ashes would be placed. We met the man in charge of cremations and a Polish man in charge of the cemetery. They were so kind to talk with us.

On the morning of the twenty-third, a goose flew by my bedroom window and honked. It was my dad. He told me that morning he had an easy transition because he'd been working on his life review for the past year. Nineteen members of our family attended the celebration of life lunch. I saw another red-tailed hawk on the way to the restaurant. I was the first one there, and I set a place for Dad with his picture, a porcelain coffee mug with a train, and a red cardinal figurine. My dad loved the St. Louis Cardinals baseball team. Don gave a nice speech. Instructions and a photo of the gravesite where his ashes would be placed in El Mirage were handed out.

My ex-husband, Hoyt, came and sat at the other end of the table. He enjoyed talking with Don, Irene, and Maureen's husband, Tom. Maureen talked with Irene. I enjoyed talking with Maureen's children,

Andrew and Amy. Amy talked about her horses. My siblings told me they missed me and that they loved me. I reciprocated my feelings of love for them. Hoyt was more prosperous now with full-time work that he loved.

I shared a memory of hiking with Dad in the Grand Tetons, taking the gondola up to the top of Mount Rendezvous at twelve thousand feet elevation. Maureen, Tom, and Val ate lunch at the crepe restaurant with Mom. Dad and I began our hike down to the eight-thousand-foot level, where we found a meadow with flowers. After lunch, we laid down on our roll pads on the ground and watched the wind blow through the aspen leaves high up in the air. I shared that when I meditated, this was one of the places I went to in my mind to relax. I could still hear the yellow leaves rapidly quivering in the wind.

Tom shared a story about Boy Scouts and how when they were hiking, all of a sudden, Dad grabbed Tom by the arm and picked him up. Tom wondered what was happening as he looked down and saw a cottonmouth water moccasin, an extremely venomous snake that delivers a potentially fatal bite, right in front of them. Dad had saved Tom's life.

Don told the story of us camping on the east coast for three weeks every summer. When we left each campsite, Dad made us kids pick up the trash, cigarette butts, and other various items, teaching us to always leave the campsite in better shape than we arrived.

We finally heard the backstory of why we called our dad Dee. Maureen said it was her who had started it, based upon reading the mail and seeing Dad's initial for his middle name, Dale, and we'd followed. It's funny how families will adopt pet names for each other, oftentimes not even questioning it.

Valerie shared beautiful memories of Dad never giving up on her. She gave credit to her loving parents. I was still so proud of her. Afterward, she and I embraced in a tight hug as she spoke to me. She cried in my arms.

Larry and I talked for a while, and he told me Valerie looked up to me and loved me. I told him I loved her, him, and all of my family very much. I had never stopped loving them, even when I was gone for those four years.

Chris stood up and shared that she always felt accepted by Dad into the family. She said he'd helped her to appreciate fine wines. When she came for a visit, and there was a meal, he made sure he had a nice wine selected for her. I looked over at Hoyt, the wine expert, and he was smiling.

After lunch, we met at my parents' home. Before I left, Andrew shared with me his sign language skills and classes. He was fully immersed in the deaf community to learn more sign language. I learned so much in that thirty minutes of listening to him. I noticed he was wearing a Star Wars spaceship design on his T-shirt. I love him so much.

Later that night, I took an Epsom salt, sea salt, mineral salt, and lavender bath to dispel the energies and replenish my spirit. I missed my father and cried into the night. I knew death was an old program that helps the human to process the abandonment wound. I knew we never die. We are eternal spirits occupying these human vessels for the purpose of ascension. To be human is possibly the greatest honor in the universe. There are humans we meet on our Earth journey that help us explore and understand more how the universe works and about our soul-purpose. As I said before, the best of the best teachers come at strategic moments in my life. One teacher with that same caliber is a man named Ronald Holt.

CHAPTER 17

Quantum Navigation Meditation

S HAMAN LANCE HEARD ASKED ME about my activities and then told me, "You need to get out of the house and have some fun."

I asked myself what I would like to do and saw an advertisement on a social media platform for a meditation group. On April 16, 2019, I attended Ronald Holt's Quantum Navigation meditation group presentation at Storm Wisdom in Phoenix. I went with no expectations. We were a small gathering of people, including Ron's wife, the lovely, amazing channeler, Lyssa Royal Holt. I admired her as a channel and felt honored to hold her in my arms with love and gratitude when we hugged. Ron was touched by my presence, which surprised me. I felt humbled. I just wanted to open my mind and heart to information I hadn't heard before or in the way Ron presented. I was curious about what he would say during his presentation.

Ron presented how the universe works, how we go through the procession of the equinoxes—into unconsciousness and back into consciousness—platonic solids, sacred geometry, our fragmentation, and much more. He used physical objects, drawings, and photos on a monitor, along with a whiteboard to illustrate the concepts he presented from his channeled information.

By the end of the evening, I felt my mind, heart, and soul had received a deep tissue massage. Very lovingly and graciously, with our minds expanding, Ron brought the newbies in the group up to speed on the concepts presented in prior months. Then, the meditation afterward was amazing. Out into the cosmos, I traveled. I shared with Ron and the group about my nothingness meditation from age seven to forty-two that I'd shared in detail in my autobiography. When I finished describing the technique, I asked Ron how the meditation fit into what he presented. With a big smile and laugh, he said it was everything he presented. Ron seemed to appreciate and know me on a level of know-ingness. He appreciated my journey and knew I'd walked the walk. People who are aware understand. We call these people in our lives "of like mind." They have gained wisdom from their experiences in life and easily recognize others who have done their inner work.

I spoke with Grandmaster Zeysan on the phone about my experience with Ron Holt's meditation gathering. I'd never told Zeysan about the nothingness meditation I had been doing by myself since age seven. After I told him the technique, he began speaking an ancient Tibetan chant. He said what I did was that chant. I then remembered that my last name with the man I was married to back in 1976 was Monk. I used to joke that I was a monk. It was no longer a joke. I had been a Tibetan monk in a prior life. Why would I know how to do that meditation at age seven? From my hypnotherapy past life regression work, I'd learned we carry skills and knowledge from previous lives into our current lifetime.

By the beginning of May, my mother was going downhill. Her brain was malfunctioning. She couldn't remember what she'd just said and couldn't hear even with her hearing aids. She had another panic attack and called me, asking if she should go to the emergency room. I went over to her house. She did have a low-grade fever of one hundred degrees, so I spent the night. We talked about moving her to an assisted living retirement community since she didn't feel safe by herself. She was sad that her life was over. She wanted to commit suicide by drown-ing in the swimming pool in the backyard. We talked about what kind of things she liked to do. She liked to watch TV and visit with friends. She didn't do arts, crafts, or games, nor had the inclination to start. The next day, she was sick with a head cold, so I went to the store and bought nutritious frozen dinners for her and a couple quarts of milk.

I called my brother, Don, and told him this had to stop. I couldn't keep running over to Mom's, and I couldn't live with her. It was obvious to me that she didn't feel safe by herself.

On May 4, she told me over the phone that she didn't want to move. The house was falling apart, and she needed someone to watch over her. She fell victim to a scammer over the phone and didn't understand how the internet works. She couldn't remember how to use her phone. She couldn't remember what pills she was taking and didn't always write down what she'd taken and when. I told her she must go to assisted living for her safety and well-being. She couldn't hear me due to her hearing loss, so I had to yell. Even so, she twisted what I'd said into something else. Trying to talk logically to her was getting frustrating, and I needed to remember that her aging brain was malfunctioning. I woke up sick with a sore throat three days later.

Zeysan sent me a text message saying the donation I made for this month to the QUESTECSS organization saved a lot of children. I was grateful, and it brightened my day, even though I felt awful from the virus in my body. The virus hit hard, and I could not work for almost three weeks. I went to the nearby urgent care center and asked for codeine syrup so I could lay down at night to sleep. I was experiencing sleep deprivation due to constant coughing. I didn't have pneumonia.

I was feeling better by May 23 and participated in Ron Holt's Quantum Navigation presentation and meditation. There were more people this time, including new people. During the meditation, I relaxed down to a deep level. I saw a scanning being done left to right to left in front of my head. I saw it as golden light. I felt an itch in my left ear and right parietal scalp, but I embraced the itch, and it went away. I found myself traveling down a convoluted wormhole. It was long, and I went out into the cosmos of deep space. When I came out of deep space, I was a dragonfly sitting on a pink hibiscus flower. I then became consciousness, traveling through space and straight into the Eye of God nebula, resting in the lower part of the "pupil." I asked for a Galactic Heritage Card and was guided to pull the Aloneness card. It was card 64, Pleiadian. All oneness—being by myself, being myself, and being comfortable in the boringness of one.

When I looked at the root wounds of the soul on the upside-down menorah, this was our journey in the Earth plane. Ron shared that we must process these attributes if we are to ascend:

Abandonment	Hopelessness	Envy
Betrayal	Nothingness	Doubt
Guilt	Fear	Worry
Powerlessness	Anger	
Worthlessness	Rage	Frustration
Helplessness	Jealousy	Irritation

Ron said my quantum navigation was confirmation of the inner work and quantum healing sessions I'd done with my clients and my own inner work in the quantum field, and the dragonfly represented enlightenment. Looking at my dream dictionary, *In Your Dreams* by Mary Summer Rain, I read that the dragonfly means a strong, positive spiritual force or aspect. The hibiscus denotes spirituality. Pink reveals some type of unrecognized weakness that can refer to one's mental or emotional state, physical aspect, or spiritual condition. The nebula was an obscure idea. The Eye of God nebula was the nothingness, consciousness, unconsciousness, and enlightenment combined.

My left lower eyelid had a minor sty, meaning a negative perception. Since this was the left side, the feminine side, it could have meant my stress about my mother and her declining health. She was in a meltdown and being sedated with tranquilizers by this time. I wanted my mom to be happy, healthy, and secure, but I knew she was grieving my dad's death.

On June 12, I asked Dolores to help me be the best QHHT® practitioner in the world, next to her, of course. She replied, "You are surpassing me. You are brave, fearless, and you don't give up on your clients. These are the hallmarks of a great QHHT® practitioner. Keep it up! Now, write this down in your book."

During the June 15 quantum navigation meditation, I saw myself sitting on the bottom of the pupil of the Eye of God nebula. I gently slipped off and went into free fall in outer space without a body, just pure consciousness. No fear, no elation, just neutral as I fell and fell. I saw a starfish and a tube torus of energy. There was flowing energy emanating from an upside-down funnel. I wanted to explore, but the quantum navigator would not allow me. Ron said that I was close into the singularity.

I drew the Galactic Heritage Card number forty-two, Pleaides, Blind Enthusiasm. The message of this card was for me to have patience, temperance, and respect for others. The Osho card I pulled was Insight. The message of this card is guidance. I was being guided. Ron told me to pay attention to the elements that showed up in my meditations.

In my third quantum navigation meditation that I did at home, I was suspended in the middle of the Eye of God nebula in lotus style, revolving to the right, then revolving upside down, right side up, and so on, in an elliptical manner.

In Mary Summer Rain's dream book, clockwise movement is said to pertain to advancement, and the gyroscope means remaining true to one's course.

I was now able to see and feel my eight years with Peter as a phase of my life, a project, and that it was also part of my mission to establish the interdimensional portal there. I no longer cried in sadness. I felt and embraced the aloneness. I moved forward on my journey, wherever it took me. "But for the grace of God, go I" was my guiding mantra.

My eighteen years with Hoyt had been a phase filled with growth, transformation, and enlightenment. His divine gift to me was to get me to strengthen myself enough to leave the nest of marriage. I would be forever grateful for his love and sacrifice for my soul's evolution. My tears were now the byproduct of my immense gratitude.

My mother was now in an assisted living facility that looked so beautiful and smelled clean. Although we had worked so hard to secure her comfort and well-being, she continued to complain. I knew this was a manifestation of her brain malfunction due to age and all the chemicals she'd ingested in the form of prescription drugs. I loved her dearly and didn't want her to suffer or be afraid. If God deemed it permissible, I would be honored to be at her side when she passed. I would coach her through her rebirth and returning home to God whenever that day came.

On June 30, during a quantum navigation meditation at home, I found myself at the Eye of God nebula. Through the nebula, I then traveled through a wormhole. The inside of the wormhole tube was green numbers and letters. I shared this with Ron, and he responded by pulling two cards for me from the Galactic Heritage card deck. The first was Seeds of Polarity, which read, "Arise when we venture away from the awesome wholeness you just experienced and be distracted into lesser perspectives." The other card was Seeking Karmic Balance, which read, "When we didn't recognize the observer as our truest self, all seeds of polarity arise in our choices and perspectives, thus we engage the wheel of seeking karmic balance."

Ron said, "You're a natural at this, Barbara, and your timing was so spot on!"

At the beginning of July, in a personal message, Ron asked me to call him on the phone. We discussed the significance of my meditation elements. His quantum navigator had asked him to incorporate what I experienced into his next presentation and told him that he must ask permission from me. I gave him permission.

I sent Ron a message after viewing his video presentation on his website titled, "Accepting and Integrating the Tempest." I had received a download of energetic information as my body shook all over but forgot to share this in the last QN meditation. It was revealed to me that I was the Eye of God nebula.

Ron responded, "Wow! You are so right about this. That was similar to the last stage before completely abiding in nothingness/everythingness. The quantum navigator gave you a stage of perspective. Now, with your last quantum navigation experience, it's signaling that it is about to take you through a number of perspective exercises to strengthen your abidance as the observer (big eye) simultaneously with source (center/singularity) and character.

"Thank you for sharing. I can hardly believe you watched 'Accepting and Integrating the Tempest!' That was one of my favorites. I accomplished the integration during a series of a few days of doing 'horse-stance' for an hour to an hour and a half each day and processing what the navigator was showing me. I find horse-stance quintessential for accepting and integrating the things we trigger and typically get overwhelmed by and thus incompletely process, and it becomes a through processing experience. I just now finished doing one hour! Again, you amaze me that you also had a similar parent and that you processed your 'Waterloo' event. I am very appreciative of your dedication to your healing and integration process, let alone your years of amazing experiences! No wonder you are having such great and profound quantum navigation experiences and are moving so quickly!"

A couple of days later, I did another meditation at home and found myself deep in a well, looking up. The sky was a medium blue. I was shown a large lotus flower made out of sparkling clear crystals, and the movement of light shone upward and outward through the facets of the crystals.

During an acupuncture treatment session, I asked the QN if it was permissible for the session to go into meditation. My Higher Self said yes. Laying on the table with Native American flute music playing, I first saw a pyramid form. I was looking down and slightly to the side of it as an observer. Then I was shown a sweat lodge, followed by a white tipi.

I received the following personal message from Ron:

Hi, Barbara. I have tailored this message below for you, and after you read it, I want to highlight what I was getting after the information foundation.

ELEPHANT TOTEM – Royalty, Strength, Honor, Stability, and Patience

The elephant is considered a symbol of responsibility because it takes great care and responsibility of its offspring as well elders. An elephant totem gives ancient wisdom and power to draw upon, embodies strength and power, and can guide you to new energies and power. Elephant people show great affection to their families (or spiritual family), caring for the young and the elderly. They also have an inborn knowledge. An elephant would give insight into the power of the three feminine energies: child, mother, and wise old woman (or crone). Elephants also express advanced sensitivity and social connection and bring a message that we are able to deal with any obstacle we are faced with. Elephants represent power, sovereignty, stability, and steadfastness. Are you remembering to nurture yourself? Elephants remind us that we must look after ourselves first before we reach out and help others. Know that we have the instincts that will lead us where we need to go and what parts of us need nourishment. Perhaps we have isolated ourselves from family and need to find our way home. Alternatively, you may have to shift your focus to view the whole picture. Occasionally, it could mean that you have to unearth buried memories and let them go.

To the Hindu way of thought, the elephant is found in the form of Ganesha, the god of luck, fortune, protection, and a blessing upon all new projects. Ganesha, in all his magnificently vibrant elephant glory, is intent on bulldozing obstacles on your behalf. Some Asian cultures also believe the elephant is a cosmic creature and carries the world upon its back, much like the tortoise does in some tribal Native American myths.

So, Barbara, the main message here was about the changes you are going through concerning the transition from Barbara the character in 3D, striving to attain a stage of enlightenment via incorporating the new vision of accepting her "Brahmic-Self," (and the self-validation, which was awakening) versus unconsciously seeking external validation for the awakening.

So, it seems that quantum navigator is attempting to stage the removal of the unconscious blocks, resistances, and any semblance of unconsciousness to further enable your self-realization to arise from within you rather than from an external perceived authority to diploma you.

This is a rite of passage in the awakening journey. It is the self-acceptance of the source within you as "the one and only Guru you have now," as no other can satiate nor validate where you stand and the new paradigm you entered. I can see it (based upon the visions you have shared), and I can validate it; however, it means nothing until you end seeking it externally and begin to sit fully within self-acceptance of it.

Yes! You have achieved a level of awakening and self-realization and go slowly now, donning the new realization while maintaining alertness for the duty of constantly remaining open to spotting, embracing, and stewarding any splits and dissociations of yourself.

Your quantum navigator points to the dragon's head you stand upon or the winged heart of awakened consciousness you possess to and nurtures any splits as they arise. You are well blessed with the tools and capacities to not only heal and awaken new levels of yourself, but by the metaphor, you are now tasked with providing it for the family that chooses you.

I sure hope this translates well and was helpful. I could write more, but I think the message essence was there. Let me know what you think or felt. Thanks again for sharing such depth and magnificent vision with me. Your gifts are amazing!

In a 4:00 a.m. dream, I saw guys shooting guns at me and others in a house, and they kept missing me. I managed to escape from the house and go to a gun store where I purchased a 9mm Glock that could turn into a rifle and then telescope back into a pistol. I returned and started shooting. The bullets traveled toward the guy, but the trajectory fell short like in the *Matrix* movie. I adjusted my focus and intention and aimed a little higher. This time, the bullets went farther and straighter. The guys who were attacking me left. No one was killed.

My interpretation of this dream was a shoot-out and a resolution of a conflict. The gun warned of mental or emotional dysfunctions, erroneous attitudes or perceptions, the potential for an emotional outburst or explosion, and may also point to a person's protective measures. At this point, I'm not sure what the warning was for. I was feeling okay, yet not always regarding my mother and her situation. The message from my Higher Self in this dream could be pointing out my emotional responses to my mother's perspective and wanting to protect her at the same time.

In August, I did another quantum navigation meditation at 2:00 a.m. in my living room. I saw colors of energy and light in gentle explosions, more like puffs, appearing in my vision. The explosions occurred in the following areas of my vision: left lower area, right upper, left upper, right lower, sides, in front, etc. I was assured by my Higher Self that this was all good.

Now, I was in the Eye of God nebula, looking outward. Then, I was shown a large white lotus flower with a dragonfly sitting on it. I realized I was the flower, the dragonfly, the stars, the space between, and everything and nothing all in the same moment. Feeling at peace and expansive, I shared this experience with Ron.

Ron replied, "Wow! Thank you for sharing that. Just magnificent! Love how your QN gave you the Eye of God nebula looking outward into creation and giving you the signs of 'all was in divine order' by showing you the white lotus with the dragonfly sitting upon it. Both powerful symbols of the flowering of enlightenment and the abiding within it. All this in addition to all the realizations concurring with it. You are accepting and validating the true self as the source and screen that consciousness moves itself as the kaleidoscopic diversity of characters and objects populate the screen. Honor your transforming and awakening Brahmin state, but remain alert. You are magnificent, and that was divine!"

The following week, I was awakened at 5:30 a.m. by the quantum navigator, and they were waiting for me. I relaxed into deep meditation and saw autumn messages. I was sitting in a home, drinking tea, and the autumn leaves were falling. I was happy sitting in the kitchen window. There was pumpkin soup on the stove and pumpkin bread on the counter. Feeling the wonderful season and inspired happiness overall, this meditation felt pleasing to me.

Autumn means a time to slow down, a time for introspection before moving on, and a natural lull in advancements. Pumpkin represents playfulness and a wide range of expressions. Soup represents a nourishing aspect generated from multiple elements. Bread represents the necessities in life and what sustains us. The kitchen represents a place of planning, clean and white. The house represents the mind, and the leaf represents natural abilities and talents. Tea represents healing strengths.

After sharing the meditation with Ron, he responded, "I was observing the last QN experience you shared while in the quantum this morning. What I got, I think you would appreciate. You have completed what you came here to do. You have seen and are consciously working and integrating whatever you have alerted your awareness toward that needs stewarding and integrating. All of which is strengthening your reconnection with your universality, leading you to be more at home in the paradox of your 'ordinariness and extraordinariness' in your daily life. You are coming home to yourself, ending any presumption while becoming confident in the notion of 'nothing to do, nowhere to go, no one to become.' Just be you, the one. It's a beautiful message of 'enjoy your time now as a universal human.' Well done!

Lance Heard contacted me because he wanted to go camping and make contact with extraterrestrial beings. We decided to go to a place we knew had rock formations of ET faces and petroglyphs of extraterrestrial beings, and I had camped there twice with the tai chi group fifteen and sixteen years ago. I'd experienced an ET in my tent the second time I went. The first time I went with the group, I slept under the stars in a sleeping bag without a tent. I had camped many times over the years with my family and independently, and Lance and I had been there and the canyon below before. We invited a client who wanted to meet ETs too.

On October 1 in the early morning, I had a dream where I looked up and saw a green frog flying through the air, doing the breaststroke. I knew this was a cosmic wink from our ET friends looking forward to Lance, Jennifer, and me camping in northern Arizona.

Lance, Jennifer, and I left to go camping on the fourth. We were in a private canyon that was accessible only by a four-wheel-drive vehicle. Jennifer's car would not make the large, high hump in the road that deterred others from traveling into the canyon. We discovered there was a large puddle from a recent rain that prevented even Lance's vehicle from driving through. We walked around the large puddle and what appeared to be a half mile to the edge of the lower canyon. This meant we had to carry all of our camping equipment and supplies back and forth from the car to the camp under the hot sun beating down on us. After we brought all of our supplies and food to the site, the wind kicked up and made the tent setup a challenge. We helped each other set up the three tents. Luckily, I'd brought my hammer, and Lance had brought his strong muscles.

We hiked down near the stream, and I was surprised to see the overgrowth of vegetation, the graffiti on the walls of the canyon, and the large pile of rocks from a rockslide where Grandmaster Zeysan had slept in his tent fifteen years ago.

I created a puja of Peruvian quartz crystals, a celestial print cloth, a white candle in a glass candle holder, and sage. I said an invocation. Lance vocalized a Tibetan chant. I played Dr. Steven Greer's meditation tones from my phone app. We invited our fellow star beings to come, stating we had come in peace with love in our hearts. We understood they could arrive and make their presence known in any way they preferred, and it was safe for them. We then contemplated in silence, looking at the stars and closing our eyes in meditation.

After about an hour, we decided to prepare for sleep. As soon as I laid down in my tent, my third eye opened, and I saw ET faces and ships. One was shaped like a faceted egg of gunmetal color, metal fabrication without seams. It hovered about two to three feet above the ground in a stationary manner. I was shown a moon type of surface, a dark atmosphere, and then the ET showed me the vector sequencing of the moon, the galaxy, and deep space.

After we moved most of the equipment and supplies to the car the next day, and Jennifer and Lance hiked up to the chimney and petroglyphs, I stayed in the upper canyon by myself. They left at 8:20 a.m. and returned around 1:15 in the afternoon. I spent the time by myself, meditating, eating, processing, peeing, pooping, and crying. It came into my consciousness that I was there to process Peter. I told Peter I was done and needed to let him go once and for all. I looked up at the side of the canyon and saw an image of Peter in the rock formation, created between the dance of light shadows and colorations of the rock formations. I said my goodbye, giving him love and gratitude to carry with him for eternity, then finally let him go.

I did not share with my camping mates that I had taken a trash bag and picked up trash on the side of the road in honor of my dad's teachings to always leave the campsite better than your arrival. I filled half of the bag with soda cans, plastic, and metal bottle caps. This was my way to honor Mother Earth and other humans who came there to visit.

I could see with clarity that the puddle of water represented emotion and spirituality, a message from Spirit that if I wanted to come, then I must walk the walk. Walking back and forth, carrying objects in and out, was part of the processing. I had bilateral tendinitis in my upper arms, limiting the amount of weight I could carry, but I realized with gratitude that I had friends who supported me and would help. I received this assistance with deep appreciation.

Lance had told his wife that this trip was important. I didn't realize how much it was important to me until it was over. On the drive back to the valley, I could feel a shift had occurred within me for the better. The following day, Sunday afternoon, the diarrhea came. I knew this was a good sign of the final release of emotions.

My cousin in New York called and told me her brother had committed suicide by jumping off the Mill Point bridge an hour from his home in Gloversville, New York. Just before driving across town to my mother's assisted living place, I delivered the news to her that my cousin David's body had been found in the Schoharie Creek in Upstate New York, the same creek she'd played in as a young child that ran next to the dairy farm she lived on. My mom knew something was wrong when I asked her to leave the bingo game and come with me to her room. When I told her that David had committed suicide, she said she'd already felt he would do something like this. From her latest telephone conversations with him, he hadn't seemed stable. David was depressed. At first, she was angry with David for taking his life. Then the shock came in. I really didn't want to give her the sad news because she was still grieving my dad's death, but it had to come from someone. I felt it would be best if it was done in person, and I was the most available at the time. I held her in my arms as she cried.

The next day, my QHHT® client offered for me to ask my own questions about my ET contact experience while camping the prior weekend. The following information was shared by the Higher Self:

Barbara: What type of vessel was the egg-shaped one, and how did it travel?

Client's Higher Self: This was an exploratory vessel with a power source that humans cannot understand. Like telepathy, not fuel.

Barbara: Do they use thought?

HS: Yes.

Barbara: Where did the ship come from?

HS: Hundreds of universes away. Not human language, like computer code.

Barbara: Did they receive my signal to come?

HS: They knew you wanted to meet them. Yes.

Barbara: Do they have a type of name that I would know?

HS: It's computer code.

Barbara: What do these beings look like?

HS: They do not have a physical form that humans can see. Not gas. Not liquid. Tiny like an atom, molecule, but complete, though small.

Barbara: Are they evolved?

HS: Very.

Barbara: Did they have a message for me?

HS: More curious. They had not come this far before. Your light was bright for them to find. They did not know it was Barbara. They knew to come to the light, your light.

Barbara: Did they recognize or understand my extraterrestrial form?

HS: Yes, but more curiosity than message.

Barbara: Did they enjoy their time with us?

HS: They will be back! They will be back when you ask. Now they know you.

Barbara: I was also shown an astronaut walking on the surface of the moon, then a vector sequencing of the Milky Way Galaxy, then into deep space. Who did that for me?

HS: It was a reciprocated message to someone you sent it to. Not to someone you deliberately meant to send it to. Someone received it and enjoyed it. It was reciprocated back as a "thank you."

On October 13, 2019, I painted three pieces of furniture and a shelf. It was hard on my body because I had to sit on concrete in various contorted positions to paint the details. As the week progressed, my right hip began to hurt, my gait became a limp, and leg spasms woke me up in the middle of the night. I made an appointment with Dr. Warwick for energy medicine and an appointment for an acupuncture session with Julie on Friday. When I went to my massage with Nicolette on October 22, I told her I wanted her to decrease the pressure by 10-15 percent. The September massage had taken five days for me to process. In other words, my body was sore, and I had no energy, even though I was drinking lots of water. Nicolette agreed.

On Wednesday, my session with Dr. Warwick was at 9:00 a.m., and I was there for two and a half hours. After each round of energy, I dove deep into theta and delta levels of consciousness, then back up into beta (awake and alert stage). Theta is just above delta, also known as sleep. At one point, I was asleep and felt someone manipulating energy over me. I opened my eyes and saw Dr. Warwick standing next to me with a smile. We finally got the range of motion to return without the pain. He pressed on my left temporomandibular joint (TMJ), and this helped greatly.

On October 24, Julie gave me an acupuncture session and said the right hip and the left TMJ area were gallbladder related. She addressed the right hip, both arms, and the right, inner elbow area. I felt much better. A Chinese medicine doctor on the other side, Dr. Wu, came forward in spirit. I spoke briefly with him. He had shown up to assist in the acupuncture session. His contribution was energetic. Sometimes he would move a needle, and I felt the pain. The pain only lasted a matter of seconds. Julie added an oil that she massaged into my right hip and leg area. The muscle fascia was very tender. She added one cupping with fire and ended with my friend, the large vibrator, massaging my hip and leg. I was purring like a kitten at the end of the session. Three days later, I was happy to report there was no more snapping in my right inner elbow. The bilateral arm tendonitis was lessening, I no longer limped, and my right hip was feeling much better.

On October 29, during a quantum navigation meditation with Ron Holt, I saw the back side of a muscular man without a shirt crawling on a white fibrous object. I then saw the world on my shoulders. I was taken to the mid-1990s when I would wake up at two in the morning with the world on my shoulders. I heard a pop in the back of the room at that moment. Then I saw a lighthouse with the light shining back and forth. The lighthouse turned into a building that looked like a fortress.

On Halloween morning between 2:30 and 3:30 a.m., I did a quantum navigation meditation in the living room, asking to dive deep into the reason or message about the panic attacks in the mid-1990s. I was shown the Eye of God nebula and entered it. I was shown a tipi entrance, and as I walk through it, I entered a portal. The sky was a beautiful blue with puffy white clouds. The environment was the Southwest desert with rock formations similar to the Painted Desert in the Navajo reservation lands. I was shown a separation as I drifted backward from planet Earth and into the cosmos. An overwhelming feeling of separation overcame me as I realized I was separating from home, the original abandonment. The panic attacks were about the impending separation from my husband. I thought back on the panic attack I'd experienced in 2011 at the ranch when I realized Peter would be returning to Switzerland and leaving me behind after assuring me he would take me with him.

On November 21, 2019, I attended Ronald Holt's Quantum Navigation meditation group. On this night, he had us lay down on the floor, and it was based on inner child healing. We journeyed backward in time, regressing before our birth. Going through the stages of pregnancy, including what we felt when our parents found out they were pregnant with us, I understood the enormous degree of responsibility that another mouth to feed represented. Everyone was happy at the birth because I was a girl, special after two boys. What was significant about this particular meditation was that I was able to experience the non-separation between myself and my parents. We merged into one beingness, one consciousness. There was more to explore. Ron's guides suggested I have a private healing session with him and my team of guides, known as the WhiteOne, and my Higher Self concurred.

CHAPTER 18

The 11:11 Code of My Enlightenment: Meeting My Twin Flame

My session with Ron Holt on November 24 was based on the inner child regression we'd done the week before in the group presentation. Lying on the Reiki table with the Moby meditation music playing, I quickly slipped into a theta level of consciousness. My nectar drops were dripping in the back of my throat so much that I asked my team to back it off a little bit because I was lying down. They obliged instantly.

Entering through a red rose in the center of my heart that became an everblooming white lotus flower, I began to journey. There were so many images, sensations, and emotions of heart love expansion and pure joy as I entered into the Oneness. At one point, Saraswati—the Hindu goddess of knowledge, music, art, speech, wisdom, and learning—was waving her arms up and down before Ron spoke her name. I smiled and went into the void. The fragments were all retracting and coming back to the center. I saw a rainbow with a white, star-shaped pulsating light in the middle and was one with it. There were times my body was hot, and others when it was cold. I felt I wasn't even on the table but suspended in the cosmos. I journeyed to my home galaxy. I traveled as pure consciousness through the cosmos. The stars and nebulas were beautiful.

I understood and felt my parents' journey, and all the facets of it were mine because I was them, and they were me. There was no separation of anything. I saw the x-y-z axis and traveled right through the middle. I saw colors of gold, blue, green, and red at various times during the journey. I cried with joy, and tears flowed from my right eye.

Ron felt the feeling of sublime equanimity and energy too. He later told me he had not done this meditation in this form before, but he went with his guides and their infinite, wise guidance, and took me through the heart. When I came out of the meditation experience, I saw everything I had experienced and wondered about, realizing that this experience explained everything. There were no more questions inside of me. I could not describe this feeling. The best I can say is that it felt like a nuclear bomb download of information from the quantum field. I truly understood and experienced the Oneness of everyone and everything.

My right hip still hurt, and I was thinking this was due to the major changes I was making in my life. I finally pulled my head out of my derrière regarding my finances. After watching many videos of Dave Ramsey, reading testimonials, and watching budget-making videos from others, I finally got it. I'd already cleared out the old programs of lack, pain, and struggle, and I felt I was a clean slate for prosperity. I figured I had at least twenty to thirty years left in my life, but if God wanted me back sooner, that was okay. However, I'd decided to make the best of whatever time I had remaining on our beautiful Earth, in service to humanity, one soul at a time.

On the 12th of December, I awoke at 2:45 a.m. and saw a cobalt blue light through my third eye with my eyes closed. Then the blue light transformed into a blue rose against the black void. I saw an ever-blooming light blue lotus flower above and to the right of the rose and knew it was time to view and experience the healing session with Ron with my eyes open.

I got out of bed, went to the living room, and sat in my meditation chair. As I listened and watched the video, the issue that surfaced was about money energy. When I returned to my mother's ancestral lineage, it was brought forth that her mother had to leave Poland to come to America, and this was a wound my mother took on when she was in utero. She felt her mother's pain of not having her mother to share in the joy of seeing and touching her grandchild. I can now see and observe with compassion those feelings about abandonment, fear of the unknown, and the death of my grandfather when my mother was two. I healed this. In the Milky Way galaxy, I saw a cat's face. In the Eye of God nebula, at the end, I saw a large rabbit. This was significant for me because years before, Quan Yin had told me my happiness was very important in my current life. At that time, she'd shown me a rabbit.

In the spring of 2020, the Covid-19 "scamdemic" occurred. Through my research and council with the WhiteOne, I determined this was a psychological warfare operation to control people and allow for the corruption to come forward for people to see. Those with comorbidities (underlying immune system disorders and disease) used the virus to transition. I believed this was the case with my mother. She was ninety years old and missed my dad very much. The virus was necessary to help more people wake up. There was more to this, but I don't want to elaborate and derail the inspirational stories in this book. I am able to see the bigger picture and know that all is in right order, and we need to go through this experience for our ascension. I will always take the positive aspect of lessons because it's all love anyway. I figure my parents went through the Great Depression. We are going through the Great Awakening.

On the 27th of April, my sister and brother, who had power of attorney over my mother, relocated my mom out of the assisted living facility to a hotel in inner Phoenix, by herself, due to their fear of mom contracting the COVID-19 virus from other residents. Within five days, my mom's health deteriorated to the point she developed pneumonia. She was taken to the emergency room and admitted to John C. Lincoln Hospital for pneumonia. Although she was treated with antibiotics and oxygen support, she died eleven days later.

In the time she was hospitalized, I arranged internet video meetings for the family so we could visit with her. My oldest brother had taken an iPad to the hospital for the staff to set up for my mom. The hospital staff would not allow visitors, even in the last hours and minutes of her death. In talking with the nursing staff on the phone, other patients who were dying were allowed visitors, but not for my mother. I will never understand why not. I do not hold animosity toward the nursing staff. I just let it go.

My mom said she enjoyed seeing us on the computer screen as we all told her how much we loved her. We told stories from our childhood so she could walk down memory lane with us. On the morning of her death, I arranged an internet video call with her, even though she was in a coma. People in comas can hear. I thanked her for the four-year project we worked on together. This was my separation from the family from 2013 to 2017. I understand it was hard on all of us. Like all things in life, this too passed.

My mother was born on a dairy farm in Glen, New York, in 1929. Her mother, Mary Slowakiewicz, immigrated from Poland to Amsterdam, New York, sponsored by her cousins. Mary babysat for the family next door during her teen years. When the mother of the next-door family died, the father, named John, fell in love with my grandmother. They married and had three daughters. My mother was the youngest child. My mother's father died of cancer when my mother was two years old. This left my grandmother with a one-hundred-acre dairy farm, raising her children by herself. She hired men to milk and tend to the cows. It was the depression, and my grandmother was poor. This left an impression upon my mother, filled with struggle, lack, and pain. I understood why my mother could never accept me having my own business and living by myself. She saw how her own mother struggled. Mom was educated in a one-room schoolhouse, graduated at age seventeen, and entered nursing school in Amsterdam, New York. My mother graduated from the three-year diploma nursing school and worked at the hospital in Gloversville, New York, where I was born. She worked as a circulating nurse in the operating room. If you ask my opinion, diploma nurses are the best nurses. Their competency stems from their training in running the whole floor of a hospital. I still hold diploma nurses in high regard.

My mom met my dad, and they were married in the winter of 1951. My oldest brother was born near the end of that year. She gave birth to four more children. She worked in hospitals in Florida and Arizona as a floor nurse. Within a couple of years, she was promoted to Administrative Nursing Supervisor at John C. Lincoln Hospital in Phoenix, Arizona. She worked the night shift and was loved by the staff and the doctors. I know this because when she retired after twenty-four years of service at JCL, she was given a farewell breakfast so the hospital staff could pay their respects. She told me that people came on their day off from work and stood in line for thirty minutes to express their love and gratitude. The medical doctors gave her a large bouquet of flowers. In my forty years of nursing, I had never seen that level of affection shown to a nurse. Because it had been twenty-six years since her retirement, no one working in the hospital in 2020 knew who my mother was. My sister made an effort to share with the staff that my mom used to work there. We know my mom felt secure and at peace leaving the Earthly plane in a place she loved to be of service for two and a half decades.

During the rest of the year, I facilitated QHHT® sessions for clients in person, without masks. Nobody became ill to the best of my knowledge. I trusted I would be supported by the universe, and that was my reality. I received an immune support liquid preparation gift from a brilliant intuitive female integrative medical doctor in Houston, Texas. I followed her instructions to drink a glass of water with the seven drops every day for six weeks. I remained healthy all year long. You read that right. It was a board-certified medical doctor. What I'd been witnessing in my practice were medical doctors transitioning to integrative medicine, finding greater satisfaction and joy in their service as healthcare providers.

One day on the Twitter platform, there was a message post with a photograph of a man kneeling in front of a machine that supplied electricity for a city in Israel. This man prayed for the electricity to be supplied for the people who benefited from it in their daily lives and businesses. I was moved by this man's thoughtfulness and generosity of blessings for people he may never meet. He also made a Twitter post inviting people to share their initials with him so he could write them on paper to place in the Wailing Wall in Jerusalem, the capital of Israel, and he would say prayers and blessings for everyone who submitted their initials. Again, I was touched by this kindness and unpretentious act. I decided, why not? I submitted my initials and expressed my gratitude for his kindness. Without my prompt, this man contacted me through Twitter messenger. He was impressed with my hypnotherapy work. I didn't respond to direct messages on the Twitter platform normally, due to the number of scam artists pretending to be friendly and honest. However, this man was different.

On September 23, 2020, Charles J. Wolfe, author of *The 11:11 CODE: The Great Awakening by the Numbers*, wrote to me through a direct message. Charlie is a regional generator specialist for Field-Core, a General Electric company, and works on power generators all over the world. His expertise is in gas, nuclear, and coal-powered generators, and his specialty is testing power generators that provide residential and commercial electricity. Charlie is a physicist with an undergraduate degree in electrical engineering and a master's degree in engineering. Currently, Charlie is working on his PhD in Applied Physics. He'd bought my book. I purchased his book and began reading.

In October, Charlie called me from Israel. I enjoyed hearing the vocal tones and feeling his energy through the sound of his voice and what he said. His communication style is sparkling, and he has a satisfying quick wit. I do have a leaning for smart men.

I was shown a past life with Charlie during a meditation. We were good friends in spirit and had worked on projects together. We agreed in this lifetime to support each other at the perfect moment. That moment was then, and we had been communicating through various platforms. I found him fascinating in every way. He insisted he was complex and difficult to understand. I found him easy to understand, given the complex situation he was in. He was going through a complicated experience and had shared his struggle on social media. We Zoomed for two hours on the 19th of October, having only meant to talk for fifteen minutes, but the time slipped away. I found his intellect, spirituality, respect, and compassion very appealing attributes in a person. Charlie wanted to come for a visit in December, and we agreed he would stay in my home office. We planned to go to the Anthem Veterans Memorial the following day.

On November 4, 2020, I received my consultation with Lisa Montgomery for feng shui for 2021. I would move some objects, add a couple more, carry a rat symbol with me, clear the energy, clean the coins, and change the container of salt in the living room corner. Lisa said a man was coming into my life next year and would become my husband. According to Chinese astrology and astrological calculations for my sign and information, marriage runs in thirty-year cycles, plus or minus five years. I was curious to see how this played out.

The Anthem Veterans Memorial was located inside a community park in Anthem, Arizona, north of Phoenix and accessed off Interstate 17. This memorial was dedicated to the service and sacrifice of our military veterans in all of the branches: Coast Guard, Air Force, Army, Marines, and Navy. There were five staggered pillars with an elliptical hole in each one for sunlight to shine through and onto a glass mosaic medallion on the ground, which was surrounded by brick pavers with the sponsored names of men and women who had served. On each November 11th, at exactly 11:11 a.m., the circular Great Seal of the United States medallion was illuminated, and people gathered to commemorate the sacrifice of our service people.

Charlie wrote about the memorial in his book because of the significance of the 11:11 code being our ascension activation number. I highly recommend his book. The reader will see how much synchronicity is playing in our lives. On November 11, 2020, I went to the memorial to join in the tribute to our country's veterans and texted Charlie, streaming the event to him. He was over-the-moon excited to be part of the event while stuck in Israel. What was significant about this was that Israel and Phoenix shared the same 33rd degree parallel location on Earth, about seven thousand miles apart. I could feel a lot of love from all of the people who attended.

On November 17, my Higher Self woke me up at 4:30 a.m. I reached over, took my phone off airplane mode, and saw several messages from Charlie. He asked me for my thoughts on his current life challenges. I texted him to call me. We spoke for an hour. I told him I would go to the Anthem Veterans Memorial that day and do a ceremony for him with Mother Earth.

Just before 11:00 a.m., I placed a beach towel on the grass on the grounds of the memorial and placed Charlie's book, a clear quartz five-pointed star crystal, a rose quartz pyramid-shaped crystal, and a goldstone made of copper filings inside glass on the towel. I went into meditation and said prayers for Charlie and all those involved in his divorce proceedings. I asked for the most benevolent outcome for all parties concerned. I then placed my hands and bare feet on the grass, sending my love and energy through Mother Earth to Charlie in Israel. Suddenly, a rush of energy came up through my hands and traveled through my entire body. It blew my mind!

The following Monday, I received a second private meditation session with Ron Holt after we talked for about an hour. My intention was to understand the interface of the Christ Consciousness, Unity Consciousness, and the Oneness in the human experience. As soon as I lay down on the massage table and my head contacted the pillow, my eyes were in rapid eye movement. I flew out of my body and into the stars. It was a phenomenal experience, as the Christ Consciousness integrated within me.

Ron Holt kindly assisted with filling in the blanks on what happened in the following account.

After the meditation, I shared with Ron about the energies I'd experienced the previous week at the Anthem Veterans Memorial. He asked if I would be willing to participate in the Eye of the Phoenix energy grid that had been established by him and Grandmaster Zeysan in 1999. I knew when we are asked to participate in sacred work, we are to accept the task. This could have meant I would have to put my book project on hold until the task was completed. And that was exactly what happened.

Ron and I met at the Phoenix North Mountain Preserve Visitors Center off of 7th Street on Thanksgiving Day. After parking, we walked the trailhead and hiked thirty minutes up on top of a smaller mountain promontory just in front of what was called North Mountain. This is where a natural energy vortex was located that Ron informed me he had nicknamed (in approximately 2009) the *Eye of the Phoenix Power Spot*. How this particular power spot came into existence was quite a story with a number of moving parts well worth recounting, as this story fits and provides valuable context in the overall construction of Ron and my recent Grid-Activation adventure.

In recounting the larger story, we have to return to the calendar date of approximately spring of 1999. While in meditation, Blackhawk—one of Zeysan's spirit guides—informed Zeysan that he was to take Ron to a location at Phoenix North Mountain Preserve. This was a different location from the Eye of the Phoenix Vortex, a spot originally created by Zeysan and used for his ceremonies. At Zeysan's power spot, he'd constructed a relatively small circle of stones denoting the actual energy vortex to which Blackhawk requested Zeysan take Ron. This site actually faces the small mountain in front of North Mountain, where the Eye of the Phoenix power spot rests but was not known to either Zeysan or Ron at that time in 1999.

Once Zeysan and Ron arrived at Zeysan's ceremonial circle of stones power spot in 1999, Zeysan enacted a short ceremony before they both immersed themselves into meditation. While in meditation, Blackhawk instructed Zeysan to take Ron to the "outlier sacred power spots" for the four sacred directions at the edge of the city, beginning with South Mountain. This was how Zeysan and Ron's adventure for creating the power spot grid around Phoenix actually began.

The outlier sacred power spots included sites at White Tank Mountains to the west, the west side of Lake Pleasant for the north direction, and Saguaro Lake for the east direction. Once ceremony and meditations by Zeysan and Ron were enacted at these four sacred power spots, marking all four of the cardinal directions was completed. Ron received instructions that a "sacred centerline" was needed for enacting a "local consciousness grid" in the form of an octahedron configuration that was needed and requested by Spirit for enveloping the greater Phoenix area within. Apparently, this was the basis for Blackhawk inspiring Zeysan to initiate Ron in the locations of Phoenix North Mountain power spots, and the outlier power spots flanking the Phoenix area were because Ron had past experience in connecting, linking, and working consciousness grid systems.

Zeysan and Ron knew that in order to connect, anchor, and activate this centerline for the entire octahedron grid around Phoenix, they needed to head on location at Casa Grande, Arizona, where an ancient, sacred power spot existed, which was created by the Ooguam Indians. This site would act as the sacred direction of the "below" for the octahedron grid while the ancient Indian site, called the Sears-Kay National Historic Preserve—approximately seventy-eight miles north—was selected for the sacred direction representing the "above."

Once this consciousness grid for the Phoenix area was activated and grounded for each site on location, and once Zeysan and Ron both shared what they'd observed of the newly created grid from their meditations, they began their daily dedication to monitor and rebalance the grid as needed.

It seemed that their meditations on the octahedral grid arose because there was significant destabilization about to occur in the Phoenix area in the upcoming periods of 1999. They both received the request from Mother Earth and Blackhawk to work together, utilizing their knowledge, heart, and consciousness on a daily basis while deep in meditation to assist this grid structure toward harmonic balance. What Zeysan and Ron practiced daily by going deep into meditation and working via instructions from Mother Earth and their personal spirit guides actually continued on for about a year. Each morning, these two shared details of their observations with each other over the phone and addressed any needed grid modifications.

Ron showed me the map he'd created and shared what was made from information he and Grandmaster Zeysan received in their dreams and meditations.

After approximately a year of monitoring and balancing the Phoenix Consciousness Grid, Ron and Zeysan both felt the work was completed, so their attentiveness to the grid gradually and naturally subsided before going dormant. That was until things changed in late 2009.

Fast-forwarding to the early days of November of 2009, Ron had been asked to assist in a national effort of Christ Consciousness Grid rebalancing with a notable group of grid workers from the east coast. The process of rebalancing and cleansing the Christ Consciousness Grid at that time was called "Djed-ing of the grid." Consciousness grids need rebalancing and cleansing as the mass of collective consciousness is constantly evolving through a spectrum of polarized consciousness states, and these states act (over time) to inculcate stratifications of dissonance, thus needing rebalancing just like a fine-tuned stringed musical instrument needs retuning on a regular basis to hold proper chords. Many notable consciousness grid shamans were being called to work together on this Djed-ing project, including Bethe Hagens of the famous Becker-Hagens Christ Consciousness Grid[31].

---

31   https://www.crystalinks.com/grids.html

Prior to November 11, 2009, Ron had been contacted by a friend named Joy, who lived on the east coast. At that time, she was in contact with many consciousness grid shamans and knew of Ron's past work in sacred geometry, as well as the article he'd written in 2003 on the Christ Consciousness Grids around the earth entitled "Sacred Geometry: The Christ Grid" by Ronald Holt and Julia Griffin.[32] Joy informed Ron of the details of the Djed project. She wanted to know if he could head to the Christ Consciousness Grid at Nodal Point UVG-17, located in Northern Mexico about eleven miles south of the Arizona border, near Sonoyta, Mexico, to assist in the Djed-ing of the grid.

Ron accepted the task but did not want to travel alone across the border into Mexico because the laws were different than in the United States, and the safety of Americans could not be guaranteed. He contacted his friend, James, who was energy sensitive. Ron felt he could be taught quickly how to sense and locate power spots and then move deeply into meditative states to work in alignment with Mother Earth and spirit guides on rebalancing the grid. Together, they parked and hiked into the rural mountain valley near Sonoyta to find the UVG-17 Grid Nodal Point within a valley surrounded by granite mountains, where quartz boulders formed a mini mountain.

Once the work at UVG-17 was completed, James and Ron returned home that evening. Ron sent in his report of the journey and their meditative grid Djed-ing observations. A few days later, he received word from Joy that the group of grid shamans determined that the Djed-ing of the grid was in need of critical additional fine-tuning; thus, Ron and James were asked to participate once again.

Neither James nor Ron wanted to risk their fate with a second venture across the border, so Ron resorted to his experiences of 1999, working with Zeysan on the "original" Phoenix Grid Octahedron Project. It was at this point that he remembered there were many power spots in the Phoenix North Mountain Preserve that could be suitably tapped into for the purpose of direct-linking with UVG-17, and he chose to use this location and Zeysan's original circle-of-stones power spot for the Djed project rather than return to Mexico. From the power spot in Phoenix and utilizing their understanding of direct links, all the

---

32   http://www.ascensionnow.co.uk/the-christ-grid.html

proposed and requested Djed-refining upgrades could easily be accomplished; thus, Ron and James set off for the Phoenix North Mountain Preserve.

On that day in November of 2009, after arriving at the Visitors Center and walking the trail toward the circle-of-stones power spot, Ron began to feel a very intense energetic sensation resembling an approximate ten-inch diameter white sphere hovering about four inches above his crown. This white, energetic sphere seemed to be instigating and motioning Ron to head up the small mountain directly in front of North Mountain, preempting the intention of heading to Zeysan's circle-of-stones vortex.

Ron informed James of this incredulous phenomenon, after which they both headed up the hill in front of North Mountain until they arrived at a clearing with rocky outcroppings that looked like perfect seats. Here, the energetic sphere moved from hovering over Ron's crown to descend into the ground a few feet in front of the rocky outcropping. Where the energy sphere went into the ground turned out to be a highly refined, beautiful power spot, and they marked the location by placing white quartz boulders exactly where the energy sphere entered the ground.

The final refinements to the grid were successful that day in November of 2009. The backstories provided enough about the intricacies of this Eye-of-the-Phoenix Vortex to understand how that links into the actual Christ Consciousness UVG-17 Grid, and it also shows how it ties into the present-day journey of Ron's and my Phoenix Octahedron Consciousness Grid adventure.

The synchronicity of repeating numbers for myself and Charlie amped up to ludicrous levels. There have been many instances of me sending Charlie a text at the exact moment he was writing my name in a text. When I look at the clock, it's Charlie's birthday numbers. The timestamps of our messages are mostly elevens. When I ordered a personalized auto license plate, specifically with the elevens, Charlie texted me to give me suggestions for a personalized auto license plate with the elevens. I didn't even tell him I was doing that! When Charlie sent me the photo of the *Matrix* license plate of the BMW at the Anthem area, the date stamp was December 11 at 11:22 a.m.

This synchronicity was beginning to bug me. Charlie suggested I had a Twin Flame reading by Dr. Harmony. He'd had a couple readings from her in the summer of 2020. It just so happened Dr. Harmony was offering a $55 discount on her Twin Flame readings, which was the year I was born! The universe was directing me into having a reading. I made the appointment. The reading was done over the internet using the Zoom video communication platform. When I showed Charlie's book to Dr. Harmony, she almost fell out of her chair with delight. A couple of interesting highlights that came from the reading included that Charlie and I *are* twin flames. Our connection was divinely orchestrated. The Anthem license plate was equivalent to shoving a memo in our face. Charlie and I were activating each other to the next level. We were also embodying all of the energy grids, Earth, human electric, and the cosmic. Dr. Harmony and I come from the same star system. My body tingled all over with chills when she spoke this information.

One important thing to remember about twin flames is that we are not necessarily meant to be physically together. Although we have cleared our karma, Charlie and I are not meant to be living together. We do our best work behind the scenes, so to speak, when we are apart, in different places on the planet. Through our individual work and through our collaboration, we activate each other's codes for ascension. Dr. Harmony explained these concepts in her book, *Twin Flame Code Breaker: 11:11 KEY CODES The Secret to Unlocking Unconditional Love & Finding Your Way Home* [33]. Her book and videos have helped me to understand the nuances of twin flames. I felt so much better after receiving my Twin Flame reading, and the synchronicity has lightened up a bit. It's very well possible that my Higher Self and Charlie's Higher Self wanted me to have a reading, and that was why they put so many signs in front of me in such a way so I could not ignore them.

Everything happens for a reason.

---

33 Dr. Harmony. *Twin Flame Code Breaker: 11:11 KEY CODES The Secret to Unlocking Unconditional Love & Finding Your Way Home*. Ask DrH Healthy Solutions, LLC, 2016.

CHAPTER 19

The Eye of Phoenix Energy Grid Work

O UR ADVENTURE BEGAN ON THANKSGIVING Day, November 26, 2020, when Ron and I met at the Visitors Center at Phoenix North Mountain Preserve. At first, he was going to take me to a different area at Shaw Butte to share a power spot, which was located at an ancient Hohokam Indigenous Indian site where spiral petroglyphs existed, denoting the many various power spots in the local vicinity. However, during a deep meditation done earlier that morning, he was told instead to take me up to the "Eye-of-the-Phoenix" power spot because I was Zeysan's student, and by lineage, I needed to have access and understanding of how these power spots at the North Phoenix Mountain Preserve came into existence.

We hiked up the shorter mountain in front of North Mountain where the Eye of the Phoenix vortex was located, then entered the circle of stone benches after bowing. The whole area was filled with white quartz rocks that Ron had carried up there during many trips over the years. He'd been instructed to fill his backpack up with quartz rocks found at the bottom of the hill, carry them up, and place them around the quartz boulders at the power spot, and the formation appeared similar to the Milky Way galaxy from above. The vibration of this area felt pulsating to me.

We sat down on the east side of the formation, and I placed a photo of Charlie Wolfe that he'd sent me from Israel. While Ron talked to me, I felt the intense energies and almost passed out, but I knew Spirit would not allow that to happen.

Ron showed me a photo of the Navajo Grandfather at age 104—who he called Chief White Eagle—and others during a visit Ron had made to see the chief. Ron opened up his backpack and pulled out a small blue box that contained the Chief White Eagle's peace pipe and Navajo sacred mountain smoke. He asked if I would join him in giving honor to the Sacred Directions and Sacred Yei-Bi-Che (Navajo Gods) as an honoring to Chief White Eagle, which I readily accepted. As Ron said a prayer and intentions, I felt a surge of energy and was suddenly connected to the grid that goes around the world. It was a definite "connection," which stirred movement inside of my physical body. I was conscious of what was happening and could see the grid through my third eye.

Ron informed me that the peace pipe he'd brought was filled with a special blend of herbs, grown and harvested from one of four different Sacred Mountains of the Navajo. Those sacred mountains include Mt. Hesperus in Colorado (I have been there twice in 2009 and 2017), Blanca Peak (also in Colorado), Mt Taylor in New Mexico, and Mt. Humphrey in Arizona. This blend, known as Night-Way Sacred Mountain Tobacco, had a higher frequency than marijuana and cannabis, so a person did not become euphoric or drowsy. However, it did enact a rapid cleansing of the mind and brought one into the heart quite quickly. This could also bring about a rapid detoxification. If one has not done enough of their inner work, detoxification can manifest instantly, with inconvenient results.

As we were smoking the pipe, I told him this smoke caused an integration. Ron was so excited I'd said that word because that morning, he'd pulled the "Integration" card from his Osho Zen Tarot deck. This blend cleansed our chakras and energy systems, left us feeling utter peace, and allowed Spirit to present what needed to be shown. Ron said a prayer, and I joined in with the mathematical star language. He enjoyed that too and took a photo of me smoking the peace pipe for the first time in my life. I then moved to another bench. Both of us facing the sun, we went into meditation for about forty-five minutes. The 11:11 Activation code of the eleven minutes after 11:00 a.m. on the clock occurred during this time. This is essential to note, as it ties in the work of Charlie Wolfe and the energy grid work we did.

I was taken straight down into Mother Earth and guided to start moving my arms in the air, making symbols such as the Mobius, and at one point, my arms were held in different directions as energy moved through my body. While I was doing this, I was being shown the planet Saturn. I said prayers for all here on Earth, plus Mother Earth. Gratitude and love were expressed from her. I saw the intersecting water flow (two converging waterfalls into the center of the river from each side of me). I dove into the water at the convergence, floating down the river to a tall waterfall. Going over the waterfall, halfway down, I emerged from the water and flew out as a golden eagle. I flew high above the landscape, then into the atmosphere, into the stratosphere, the ionosphere, and out into the cosmos, out to the beginning, the end, and the beginning of All That Is. Out there, I was shown a beach with the ocean water spreading out on the shore of love. All was love. I was completely immersed in love. It was blissful.

Ron later shared that his meditation had him experience all of the anguish and polarizations of the Phoenix collective consciousness that was currently mirroring the collective consciousness. It came about from the heightening of dissonance on Earth as we faced the changes in the astrological influences, as well as the ascent in the galactic 26,000-year cycle, crossing the midplane and returning into the feminine reintegration cycle. He worked with it until he felt a balance.

As we hiked back down the mountain, Ron showed me the mountains to the north that surrounded our valley, saying they were approximately 1.7 billion years old. Over time, they had crumbled and filled the valley with two thousand feet of lava rock.

On November 30, I wrote an email to Ron informing him that I had dreamed of riding on a motorcycle with Zeysan toward Casa Grande, Arizona. Zeysan was driving with no shirt on. I could feel his belly. Then I was sitting outdoors at a picnic table with others. I looked up into the blue sky, seeing light codes and ET craft zipping around. To my right, I saw Mother Earth flying behind us on a trajectory orbit and wondered to myself, *If that is Mother Earth, where am I?* I looked down and saw the lunar surface.

Ron felt the dream messaging not only validated but necessitated taking me to each site of the grid. He said a shirtless Zeysan connoted transparency and vulnerability and that we both would need to act out each stage and chapter of this shamanic process we were about to take from a state of ultimate vulnerability, which was a form of surrendering to the unknown first. This form of surrender was true shamanism, as it was not mechanical in ritual and was actually beyond ritualism. In this depth of vulnerability without personal will and ego, each phase of this project could be orchestrated by Spirit through our naked vulnerability and transparency.

However, unbeknownst to me at that time, in his early morning meditation on the same day of my dream about Zeysan, Ron received that the previous day's venture with me at the Eye of the Phoenix Vortex, during his meditation, had exposed a window into experiencing the level of dissonance arising in the Phoenix Consciousness Grid simultaneously with the national and international grids. All of which resulted in Mother Earth making a request. Mother Earth requested that if Ron and I were willing to commit to reactivating and then balancing and monitoring the Phoenix area grid, then she would guide and assist.

However, Ron did not inform me that he'd requested of Mother Earth a very clear sign that I (Barbara) was the right choice and capable of the commitment. So, when I wrote to Ron about my dream of riding on the back of Zeysan's motorcycle, this actually confirmed for Ron by Spirit that this was right. He then proposed the offer to me of reactivating the former Phoenix Octahedronal Consciousness Grid.

Ron slowly began revealing more of the grid, its locations, and past purposes. It was at this point that we became united in purpose, so we both shared all of the signs we received from Spirit while remaining in as open, vulnerable, and transparent a state as possible with each other. I felt an immense honor and responsibility to Mother Earth and humanity to participate in this grid work to the best of my ability, in whatever manner unfolded. Our schedules opened and coincided for the grid reactivation project to begin with the ceremonial activation of the Casa Grande Ruins.

Ron and I drove to Casa Grande Ruins and performed a ceremony to close the old energies and open the new ones. Because the state park was quite open and there were visitors milling about, he felt there was no privacy to enact a sacred ceremony, so we resorted to smoking the peace pipe in his car for the personal cleansing and preparatory setting of the necessary intentions and prayers. Once completed, our intention was to proceed out to the power spot itself to enact the ceremony.

Once we walked out to the Casa Grande ancient ruins, Ron retrieved two tiny pieces of silver from his pocket to place in the adobe house for part of the ceremony. He shared with me that in Navajo tradition, silver was a gift to be given, representing and respecting the Yei Bi Che (God) that holds the sacred direction of the below. We saw a white feather on the ground in front of the Grande house, which was a positive sign for me. Ron informed me that next to the Grande house ruins was an additional power spot. He wanted to check and verify if it was to be used, but he quickly decided that it was of insufficient intensity and did not feel right. At the sacred power spot at Grande house, I noticed it helped open my heart chakra even wider than it already was.

We sat on the base of one of the pylons for the large canopy that covered the house ruins, which was constructed in order to protect Casa Grande from the elements. Ron channeled Grandfather Chief White Eagle, and I moved my arms in the air, making symbols, moving energy, and began the mathematical star language. The WhiteOne came through in the masculine side and spoke a message for us. We did not record this.

Ron enjoyed the channeling, then went on to place the silver into the back wall of the house. I went inside to see and be in the house, anchoring my energy to the interior. After the channeled messages, I felt compelled to inform and show Ron that I was guided to bring a small stone as a gift with me, which was called goldstone. Goldstone is made of copper filings inside glass made of silica and quartz.

When he saw it, he lit up excitedly and said, "This is another sign from Spirit, as you could not have known prior to this that 'gold' is the Navajo symbol of the Yei Bi Che (God) of the sacred direction of the 'above.' I was not intending to ceremoniously activate more than one site today. I was going to wait for the appropriate sign, but you just provided the sign, and this was so serendipitous that I cannot help believing this means we are to place it today in the power spot designated for the 'above' point of the central pole, which is up near Castle Hot Springs/Lake Pleasant area. So, if your schedule is open for it, we can head out now and perform it."

I told Ron my schedule was wide open, and we decided to go to the feminine point straight from the Casa Grande Ruins.

Ron had not returned to that sacred "above" point since he and Zeysan had first activated it. He could not remember exactly where it was located but was confident that the power spot energetics would signal his senses when he got in proximity to it. We had to resort to using our extra senses and intuition for pinpointing the exact or near-exact spot. The drive was over ninety-seven miles north.

As we drove just west of the Lake Pleasant area, we saw two bald eagles circling in the air. As we passed by a hill, we could feel the strong yet refined energy on our crown chakras. This sensation dissipated as we continued driving on the dirt road, away from Lake Pleasant on a back road. We also saw a red-tailed hawk in the air. Then Ron pinpointed a particular volcanic mountain, and his senses validated its appropriate significance. We resolved to drive the current dirt road to get as close as possible to the volcanic and energetic peak.

As we neared the peak, the road had taken a direction down and up a steep embankment. Ron could not get his four-cylinder, front-wheel-drive vehicle to go fully all the way up the hill, so we left the car at the bottom and hiked up to a clearing. At this clearing, the energies we experienced heightened. Additionally, we saw a red cardinal on a branch of a Palo Verde tree that seemed to accentuate the sacredness of the spot we'd chosen for the anchoring ceremony. We selected a spot that was also next to a tall, sentinel-like standing saguaro. Sitting down, we could see the lake in the distance, and the sky was a beautiful pristine blue without any clouds. Together, we caught our breath, centered, then smoked his peace pipe in preparation for the ceremony.

After a beautiful invocation by Ron, I channeled the mathematical star language, very soft and feminine this time. Toning came through, and Mother Gaia came forward to give us a message. Ron said Grandmother showed up just before she spoke through me. He really enjoyed the experience, as I did too.

Ron took my photo standing in front of one of the sentinels, saguaro cacti that are straight and tall. He took my goldstone for burial. While pouring the pipe tobacco mixture over the goldstone and into the hole he'd made, Ron blessed the four directions.

When this part of the grid work was complete, we walked back down to the car. When we got to the part of the road that was very steep, about a 45-degree angle, we could not get the car back up the road and had to walk up to the main dirt road at the top of the hill. I offered to call the Arizona Automobile Association road service (AAA) since I had cell phone coverage. Ron agreed. It took AAA forty-five minutes to determine they could not help us since we were on a dirt road. This was my first time calling this service for an off-road situation. During that time, Ron told me about how he and Lyssa met. It was a wonderful and magical story filled with humor and intrigue.

There we were, standing in the desert, seeing cars in the distance travel a road that went to Lake Pleasant. At one point in his story, Ron said, "Barbara, this is a long story." I replied, "Well, Ron, I hate to break up the fun here, but I have got places to go and people to see." We doubled over in laughter, considering we were going nowhere fast.

Ron left me to flag someone down, and as he walked away, I said to myself, *There goes the masculine taking action.* I felt perfectly cared for, supported, and not alone while standing in the desert. I did not even care if Ron never returned. If this was how I would leave the Earth, then so be it. I was in total surrender. Perhaps this was our test of not stepping into fear and instead choosing to enjoy the experience.

Ron returned about ten minutes later with an older couple driving a Ford 250 truck with a camper shell. The man had a strap for towing, and the couple drove down and hooked up the car. It was getting cold up on the hill. I decided to sit on a large rock that looked like a bench, closed my eyes, said a prayer, and went inward. I said out loud, "Let's see what happens next." Within a couple of minutes, I heard the vehicles coming up the hill. For humor, I stood up with a smile with my right thumb out like a hitchhiker. We thanked the couple. I obtained their names and address so I could send them a Christmas card and money for their effort, time, and energy. The total time we were "stranded" was ninety minutes.

During our drive back from this day's hilarious events, Ron informed me that he was attempting to decipher whether we were to initiate the opening and anchoring of the four cardinal directions of the octahedron beginning from the direction of the east (as was the traditional directional opening), but since Spirit was in charge of the orchestration and construction, we were to await its signs to proceed and surrender all attempts to control the orchestration of events. We both hoped we'd receive something soon.

On December 7, I had a dream where I was on the motorcycle with Zeysan again, but this time, he was wearing his black tai chi uniform. His long gray ponytail hung down in front of me. We went to the Cave Creek/Carefree power point at the Sear-Kay Ruin. Since we didn't know which power point to activate next, I asked in my dream, "How do we know for sure that this is the first one to go to?" I saw a pyramid of light with transparent sides. Just the edges of the four-sided pyramid were lit up, and the entire shape was placed over the area. I took that as confirmation.

I shared the dream with Ron, and he said our work had been acknowledged and formalized. Congratulations to us both. We'd passed the test, so to speak. We agreed to go to the north power point on December 8.

Ron wrote to me, "Impromptu dream work prompting today's northern gateway power spot ceremony for December 8th's alignment (Pallas Athena moves to Aquarius on December 8). The warrior goddess opens the door to Jupiter/Saturn. Aquarius. Athena was the virgin, meaning she remains true to her origins outside the Earthly realms and remains ever in her goddess form, untainted by man or mortality. She was born fully formed from the head of Zeus. So, the north was pointed to the void and the goddess, so we begin the four cardinal direction ceremonies by the north, thus opening the vessel (octahedron) to that of the Goddess. This ceremony is in conjunction with December 4th's Casa Grande alignment and ceremony. So incredibly beautiful and humbling."

I added, "This is also December 8th, the Feast of the Immaculate Conception. The conception refers to the divine feminine."

On December 8, Ron and I drove to Sears-Kay Ruin in the North Cave Creek area of Arizona. We were alone. We asked permission of the people of the land who had lived there before we ascended the mountain, then hiked up to the top of the native ancestral home. We could see the Four Peaks Mountain and Weaver's Needle rock formation in the far distance. Brother wind was with us because it was very windy, causing the wind chill factor to be appreciated. For me, this was the most powerful point of the grid so far, besides the North Mountain center point.

The Sear-Kay Ruin was built by the Hohokam tribe in 1050 AD, and it had been abandoned around 1200 AD for unknown reasons. In 1887, J.M. Sears established a ranch in this area, and the ruins were discovered by soldiers of the 5th Cavalry Regiment out on patrol from Fort McDowell. The ruins consist of forty rooms. In September of 2020, a wildfire destroyed most of the vegetation of the site and surrounding area. Ron and I saw the blackened hillsides from our vantage point at the ceremony.

While Ron gave the invocation, he named the obsidian arrowhead as an honoring of the north's association with the void and used charcoal dust to honor the covenant and guardians of the north. I held the onyx arrowhead in my hand, then transferred it to my heart between my breasts, inside my bra. I connected to the Earth's grid and to the cosmic grid. We smoked the peace pipe. I channeled the mathematical star language. The WhiteOne came forward and gave a message and blessings to us. Grandma Chandra (Chief Golden Light Eagle of the Ihanktonwan Band of South Dakota was her grandson in a previous life) appeared in the form of her Ascension app suddenly showing up on my cell phone. We sat for a while after the invocation and allowed Spirit to move through us while we remained in meditation.

During meditation, the ETs and ancestors were present with us. Everything was connected, and I felt completely one with All That Is. Coming back into my body was profoundly elegant and slow. We saw a black raven land on the large rock below us known as the "Rock Jug." A red-tailed hawk circled above. Ron was able to photograph the hawk. It was awesome! During the channeling, a bee landed on his hand. It was very windy and cold up there, but our hearts were warm with love, gratitude, and humbleness. We were told there would be more instruction. I sent photos and a brief report to Zeysan. He replied, "I love that place."

Ron and I were understanding more that we were of Zeysan's lineage, in that we were Tibetan monks in a prior life. We are students of his tai chi and his wisdom in this life. Ron said it would take a powerful woman to bring in these new energies coming together as the Pallas Athena, and it would take many others to anchor in the octahedron and close the old energetics installed by the former energy grid architects. Ron intimated that it had to be a woman—or a man and a woman—working together in absolute harmony because the masculine was behind us. Now, it had to be the integrated sacred union of the feminine and the masculine. This information coincided with the information I'd received from the Native Indian elders at the Star Knowledge Conference I attended in Carefree, Arizona, in December 2012. The eight hundred participants at that conference were told to be strong going forward because it was going to be very rough on planet Earth as she and her children evolved. We were the ones who would comfort those awakening to truth out of the matrix. Would you agree they were spot on for 2020?

After we completed this ceremonial process and were headed home, Ron informed me that it made sense that the north cardinal point was selected by Spirit in leu of the coincidence of the Pallas Athena portal opening, but he was perplexed in determining if the east cardinal point was the next ceremony, or if it should be the west and the start of a counterclockwise ceremonial procedure used when matters are to move toward Spirit and off the planet. The motion toward counterclockwise made sense if we were reversing, so to speak, the past patriarchal and clockwise motion of ceremonial activation.

Guess we would need to see what Spirit had chosen. We needed to watch our dreams and visions carefully over the next few days and go from there.

Charlie Wolfe arrived in Phoenix on December 9, 2020, and we talked until about 9:00 p.m. He slept in my healing/hypnosis office after we enjoyed a pot roast dinner with rolls from the Spicery restaurant and a 2017 Cabernet Sauvignon called Le Pich. Le Pich is French and means "golden eagle." The wine from Purlieu Winery was very good.

In my meditation that evening, I saw two white quartz pyramids pointing to each other in a vertical manner. When they moved toward each other, there was a burst of white light in the middle. I shared this image with Ron.

On December 10, in another meditation, I saw an engineer's compass, a clock face set at 11:00, the letter Z, and an image of a uterus with ovaries that morphed into the zodiac sign for Aries. The Aries sign was eaten by a fish.

On this same night, Charlie and I went out to dinner at Tandoori Times. He gave me a cashmere shawl that I wore to the restaurant. We enjoyed a variety of Indian dishes consisting of a very hot, spicy chicken vindaloo, a mild mater paneer chicken biryani, garlic and onion naan (my favorite), a vegan patty called Aldo Nikki chole, and two pastries called samosas chole. The food was delicious, and we returned to my apartment with leftovers to enjoy the next day.

The following morning, we went to the Anthem Veterans Memorial to take photos and feel the energies. He made a video with me in it, and we had our photos taken together at the memorial by a fellow visitor. On the way back to the apartment, I momentarily stopped at the red light, forgetting I could turn, then realizing I could turn right on red about the time the light turned green. That was not like me. As I drove on Daisy Mountain Road toward Interstate 17, a white BMW M4 moved in front of me with the license plate 11011, fully customized with a *Matrix* movie background of green vertical rows of ones and zeroes. "Barbara! Look at the plate!" Charlie exclaimed, taking photos. Both of our jaws dropped. This would be the most profound sign of our time together. It felt like a cosmic nod that we were to be in that location, together at the same time, and that there was significance to the event and the energy activities we were engaged in.

Since Charlie was here, he would participate in the ceremony with Ron and me. Ron picked us up at 2:15 p.m. on Friday, December 11. On the drive to the White Tanks Mountain State Park, Ron explained the grid and the energy work we were doing. He said that after reviewing my meditation download and from his own morning meditation, he'd determined that the White Tanks power site with its waterfall was the next ceremony to do viewing and that the west, in Navajo, was the direction of the Pacific, which was water and the mineral turquoise. I enjoyed sitting in the front passenger seat, listening and watching the show as these two men conversed. I truly felt I was both of these men. Their voices were beautiful music, and I felt the Oneness. There was absolutely no separation. I felt Ron's oration of the grid work, and Charlie's input was interesting for us to hear because, from this, we could learn a lot about the ascension of humanity. Here's a bit of that conversation:

> Ron: What we were trying to determine was whether we were to go right and or left hand counterclockwise, moving the grid activation toward Spirit or clockwise to work with harmonizing physicality. We suspected it was going to be left hand, counterclockwise, because it was time to move the old grid back into Spirit. Now, Barbara, you sent me the image with the two pyramids you saw in your meditation. It's a model that was the engine for creation. That is when you have yin and yang. In order to have creation, you have to have yin and yang and the DNA from both in order for physicality to take place. So, this aspect, what we were trying to do since this is the Pallas Athena opening the grid with the feminine—the unstructured feminine, and then catalyzing itself into the grid—that was the symbol of the unification of those two coming together, which was what you saw in your meditation.

> If you look at any creation model, you'll see this portrayed as two triangles pointed toward each other, which was also depicted as a side view of a spiral from a wide toward narrow turns in one way like a triangle pointing toward a spiral turning the opposite way, starting from a narrow to wider turn, creating a side view of an opposing triangle.

> These two triangles—or opposing spirals—form a torus field, and inside of this torus field was manifestation and creation. So, you have the two opposites inside the torus structure, which also repeats outside the structure.

On the Earth and during our sojourns in the body and within society, the pyramidal shape symbolizes the consciousness that has been evolving throughout the patriarchal archetypes of logic, reason, law, and order—all contributing to understanding the strengths and weaknesses or pros and cons of structure, all developing over time that pyramidal shape of experience of life.

It is this symbolic pyramidal experience. When merged with the strengths and weaknesses or pros and cons of archetypal feminine unstructured experience, that directly leads to awakening and only happens when we are mature in experience to have them come together without their propensity for combating or competing with each other.

We have been asleep. This is how all of this has started. We volunteered to go to sleep in order to wake back up to and entertain new possibilities, new probabilities. Right at this time, we are facing the 2012 crossover of the galactic median, and that was supposed to be the Mayan point that denoted we were coming back from underneath the galactic disk. It was where we experience the thirteen thousand years of unconsciousness, and it was one-half of the galactic processional cycle of twenty-six thousand years.

We are crossing the midplane of the galactic disk, so we have been transitioning slowly from externalized creation and the pursuit of identity and resolutions from an externalized perspective, which means "something out there can fix me, and I must find it out there."

Now that we are entering the Age of Aquarius, for those who are ready and those who are doing their shadow work and integrating it and refusing to project unconsciousness on others, these are the individuals most able to accept their full divinity and bridle it, really sit within it. Then, that is the Age of Aquarius.

Because they have got the full awareness, full consciousness of the experiential separation realm and the divinity it hones all together as one—masculine, feminine, divinity—all unifying together in compassionate understanding, appreciation, and clear-seeing.

Charlie: So, what you're saying is not everyone is going to wake up on December 21? Each one wakes up individually?

Ron: Succinct. Right on!

Charlie: I think the same thing about Christ. I think Christ's returning is an internal chemical process that takes place when someone is punished enough, that has been down deep enough to the lowest of low situations. Right?

Ron: You're *awesome*! Yes, yes!

Charlie: You get pounded and pounded. Then you take your T shot. The joke is the punchline, right?

Ron: Yes, yes. And the tempering. You go through all the tempering of the shadow, and then you start to integrate. Nothing—*nothing*—is not divine! So, it all has to go back, but we can't have a judgment on it. We have to see why it's divine.

Charlie: You and Barbara are drinking from the same cup because this is what she was saying yesterday. I had a hard time with it, but it's making better sense today.

Ron: So, that symbol that you had been given, Barbara, of the two triangles pointed toward each other. On many different levels, it is acknowledging the work that we did. We already set the above and the below energy pole at Casa Grande and the power spot by Lake Pleasant. Then, we opened up the cardinal point north gate. We have two alignments that are commonly placed into—when they build cathedrals, those cathedrals know of the great conjunction.

Charlie: Was this like ley line type stuff?

Ron: Yes. So, in these cathedrals, you have to look closely, but you will find the St. George and the St. Andrew's crosses. These crosses denote— It depends on how you look at it, but you can say the earth is the primary north, south, east, west.

Charlie: But in terms of universal perspective…

Ron: In terms of the universe, it's not! The universe is the great cross. The Earth is on the X. So, when the X and the cross line up, that's supposed to be the conjunction. You need to know those two when your (Barbara's) dream element came into place. The cardinal compass and the universal. Well, in this case, the cardinal compass was showing the universe what time. Because the universe keeps its own time, right? The solar goes between—

Charlie: The astronomical years, that kind of stuff?

Ron: Yeah! Perfect! So, in the earth, we go through the period of the masculine, which is total separation consciousness, and then it's got to move into integration consciousness, which is the feminine and unstructured consciousness. So, this era that we are in now is starting to align back into galactic alignment. That's when the X and the Y come into unison. If you're ready, then you'll start to feel your universal order and beingness coming in. Right? You didn't listen to the markers of the hierarchy that be and the old external navigational points, which are feeding the ego. We are all switching to what feeds our soul, spirit, and consciousness as navigational markers.

Charlie: I got you.

Ron: But in order to not listen to the orders of the hierarchy that be, you have to understand deeply that the hierarchy that be are Saturnian. Who is Saturn but us? Saturn creates the laws, the architecture of society, like protocols, rules, regulations. That's all Saturn. The administration and adjudication of those laws, we have to experience standing in that role, but because we're both doer and victim and rescuer, especially during the separation consciousness where everything seems like "It's them, not me," eventually, you come to the realization that everything is a reflection of you.

In order to understand the divinity and structure, you have to understand that without the structure, all there would be is a bunch of damn thugs all vying for power and control from a basis of entitlement.

Charlie: The geometry, at the most fundamental levels, all comes out in geometry, in mathematical order so that it can be observed.

Ron: Yes! So, when you're at the experiential level where you're okay with knowing, yeah, I have been both male and female in how many different lives, that eventually leads to acknowledging and accepting that actually I have been both adjudicator of the law and have also had to herd the cats, so to speak. Keep them in line! [laughing] But also, you're the cat, always seeking freedom. You have been both parts through this entire separation journey and the many lives it generated. So, when you're appreciative and feel on a deep level, because of all your acknowledged experiences of past lives and positions with their many belief systems you have held in past lives, you intimately and personally know the pain that it takes to follow an order coming from a seemingly unfeeling, sterile, and clinical Saturnian patriarchy.

Eventually, you come to the point of realization that the only authority there is, is you and Creator. [laughing] You have to go through all of that because you follow the lead of the group, the peer group, the societal group, the national group, the world order, so on and so forth, until you become conscious again. There's a greater order, and now I am standing up for that. That's kind of the cross and the X coming together, an opportunity, a graduation moment. Are you ready to own all the lifetimes you were in and see compassionately how you are now?

You are both the grid, the architecture of authority, rules, regulations, models of behavior, to the point where, like in martial arts, you learn all the rudiments until you are at that mastery level. Go ahead, throw anything at me. My body is ready. Just do it. That's the divinity you stand on. It's very light to stand in that kind of divinity. Then you set the operation. You change how rigid the structure is, how rigid Saturn is. You're ready for Jupiter, expansion. You're free to move about the cosmos or the continuum because you've learned the rudimentary lessons. You're almost like a self-guided policeman, except you don't have to wear a badge and a star. You have so much compassion and understanding and experience. I know how you feel when someone is robbing you of your rights or too much authority, manipulation, or control.

Charlie: Time to break the system. Whom do you get your orders from? How do you get your instructions?

Ron: Well, I need to explain. So, this is the graduation point, but as we awaken, it has to be a self-invitation. When you awaken, then you have the right to go to any of the power points in the grid system and modulate it according to the divine. You move, and you take your orders from a much higher, universal consciousness. You moderate it, getting it ready for the new. All those who have graduated didn't need this manipulative, sterile, over-controlling, micromanaged… When you feel it, then you are ready to move. They just guide you. "Go here and do this." So, you move in coordination with that, and they show you what to do. It's done mainly from the inner heart maturity.

Charlie: Okay.

Ron: Now, that compass thing (engineer's compass) is brilliant because it's denoting these two factors. You could not have known that. That is awesome that it came in! Again, we were wondering if it should be left hand or right hand.

Barbara: And I was feeling to go to Saguaro Lake, but no, I was still open [to which power point to go to].

Ron: The morning before Barbara wrote to me, I was in the quantum, and all of a sudden, they were showing me, "Go here." Like where we are going now. Like in Chinese five element theory. Everything came from the quantum. The quantum is a fluid. It is the most inclusive of all fluids. If you take the pH out of water, it's called universal solvent because everything dissolves in it. Quantum fluid is the fluid medium that everything comes back into. The consciousness is so inclusive that it's fluid, and it's so loving. Everything pops up from the quantum in equal opposites.

Charlie: Complex conjugates.

Ron: There you go!

Ron and Charlie laughed.

Ron: In the five-element theory, water came first, like the quantum waters, and out of that came fire and light. Next came earth, followed by wood, metal, and then back to water. In Western five element, it depends on how you want to associate it. It's fire, earth, air, water, and ether. They rotate opposite each other. To understand why they wanted us to go here first and then over to the sun, you have to go into the element theory. Everything in the quantum is in such perfect balance and peace. Nothing has to manifest because yin and yang found a home in each other, so they disappear just as every equal opposite does. So, that quantum fluid, it's an ocean of equal opposites. This ocean is so relaxed and neutral inside of itself. It's so at peace, and so at bliss, "Oh, I didn't want to manifest. Oh, forget that!"

Charlie, Ron, and I all laugh together.

Ron: Yet, the quantum is pregnant and ready to manifest, like a spring ready to uncoil and spring out, but something has to instigate it to do that. So, they represent that as fire. Once fire comes along, then quantum diversity springs out and creates what the ancients called the ten thousand things, but obviously, it is a lot more than that. That's what is understood as being quantum water. So, the wood and the earth create the living things. Wood represents all the green and living structures and living nature. Then its metal, which attracts water again. That water is different from quantum water. So, understanding of that five-element theory, we went from opening the Pallas Athena gate, which caused the connection, so they were acknowledging "You did it!" That Athena energy of the divine feminine, which was unstructured, was fierce consciousness. She is divine, unstructured consciousness.

So, that night, I had a dream, too, of an immaculate white owl. And that's her [Athena's] signet. The owl is also the Goddess Saraswati's signet. She rides the back of the owl. So, that was a good indicator that we did it. We cocreated its opening, and now they want to invest that by grounding it into the water as a beginning. So the west, as I said before, in Navajo, it is equated with the ocean and represented by the color turquoise.

Barbara: Look at us! We are all wearing turquoise shirts! The three of us put on shirts with varying shades of turquoise! This was done unconsciously, therefore divinely! [We laughed.]

Ron: That unstructured female, Pallas Athena, is being invited into the water structure of the planet. The next cardinal point and gate to ceremonially open after the west/water is that of the fire. Fire is mind. Fire is Aries. First, it's got to go into the water. That's what we are doing today. So, do you see just how phenomenal that the guidance is? Just, "Go here, and then, go over there." It must first be anchored in the water, which is also the emotional body for the entire planet. After the water, knowing five elements, it goes to the mind next, where the new energy sets the lattice works for letting the mind settle. When the mind settles, then it becomes the receptacle for consciousness. So, that's the next step.

When the mind is still, it becomes that perfect clear sphere, like a pond that is absolutely still. You can see and feel everything. The feeling of the quantum has to spread to the mind, and then it starts to settle. Then next, we go to the south, which is the physical, the earth. So, we ground it into the physical and the earth.

Charlie: This goes back to the biblical allegory of the symbology of the Israelites being lost in Egypt. That's the lower part of the body. It's the lower parts of the body that function that got stuck in the first forty years of life. Then, you get back to the Promised Land, right?

Ron: Yes! Yes! You're awesome!

Charlie: We're reading off the same sheet of music, brother!

We all laughed.

Barbara: You guys just click! I just knew it! Ron, Charlie's very brilliant. He's very empathic and a very compassionate person.

Charlie: That's true of everybody in this car right now. You guys just have a few years on me. I didn't get into this spiritual stuff until about four years ago.

Ron: Oh really? Well, obviously, you've done it in past lives because it's coming back like mad (very fast).

Charlie: Over in Israel, I was working at 32.6° north of the equator, which rounds up to thirty-three. I was right next to ancient Phoenicia. And here I am today at the 33rd north parallel, also named Phoenicia. I am going through a bad divorce right now and here to rebuild from the ashes of being three months by myself and dealing with that divorce. Two weeks of solitary quarantine and stuff like that. I am here to rebuild the bird from the ashes. Energetically, it's a good timing thing for me.

Ron: Oh my God! This is so appropriate.

Charlie: That's why I wanted to bring these rocks with me from the Dead Sea.

Barbara: And this was where you wrote my name in the sand?

Charlie: Correct.

Ron: Well, we would certainly use them. This one may be perfect for the next one. I certainly can empathize with what hardships you are going through and your clarity to use it as a honing and pruning process of integrating the shadow within. I have gone through quite a number of similar such ordeals in my life. My father died when I was eleven. I watched my mom for two weeks, sitting on the rocking chair and balling her eyes out. She could not do a darn thing. I credit my mom for her actions in that chair, allowing all the pain and grief out before moving on and teaching us how to handle extreme tragedy.

When I was twenty-one, I was to be married to the love of my life, but she died tragically in an auto accident, which really threw me for a loop for the next ten years. Have you ever seen someone who dies quickly, how their skin turns that ashen color? When she died, I was at my best man's house, as we were only a week away from getting married. I felt a terrible trembling inside and went to go find my fiancé. I went up the road, and sure enough, it was her car in an auto accident.

I went to the morgue where her body was, and when I saw her, her skin was very alive. I knew she was still there and sat with her for a while, said my goodbyes. For the next ten years, I felt soul-crushed. I would go out to the forest and ball my eyes out. Then, Spirit would come. I also would go into empty churches and ball my eyes out just like I remembered my mom did in her rocking chair after my dad died. I got very sensitive to energies. Little did I know that I was developing my relationship with Spirit and being taught not to attach or hang onto anything.

Eventually, I started the Flower of Life, which is an organization based on sacred geometry. You can find information on the sacred geometry from the book, *The Ancient Secret of the Flower of Life, Vol. 1 and 2* by Drunvalo Melchizedek. They are good to read. He gave me the organization, so I ran it for seventeen years and gave it back to him in February of 2013.

Charlie: I think I have that book.

Ron: That's where I got some of my sacred geometry.

Charlie: That's crazy cool!

Ron: Yeah, then there's my wife, who is an author. Her field of expertise is in all of the galactic connections. She writes on UFOs and ETs and their galactic history.

Charlie: If you told me this four years ago, I'd have told you all of the people in this car were more looney than fruitcakes. Nuttier than squirrel shit.

Ron and Barbara laughed.

Ron: Now this stuff is starting to make sense!

Charlie: It's starting to snap together. If you start to pull away enough layers of the lies, you start to see the truth of everything.

Ron, Charlie, and I walked up the path to the waterfall area of the park. It had rained the night before, after Charlie and I went out for dinner, and there was a small collection of rain in the depression in the rock formation. We waited a while for the number of tourists to diminish; however, people kept coming to the area. Knowing this was Spirit showing up for the ceremony, we found a small nook aside from the pathway where others walked, and Ron began the ceremony.

Ron: We will bring our attention to the heart space. That heart space is actually the singularity. Each of us exists as a singularity. Singularity is the consciousness, the universe, galaxies, and even the void itself. All is brought about into manifestation by the singularity. So, we are bringing our awareness and attention into that peace—center of our being, center of our consciousness, center of our heart. As we do, we set the intention to invite the presence of the Great Mother, the heart of Mother Earth. Yes, her presence and participation, interaction, and assistance in this sacred ceremony of activating, intentionally bringing our awareness and attention first to the center of the North Mountain grid point, Eye of the Phoenix.

Next to the sacred Above and Below, we honor the Yei bi Chei with this mineral silver and gold as we invite those present, anchoring in the above and the below. From there, we consciously connect from that North Mountain Eye of the Phoenix, connecting the intentional sacred geometry consciousness connections directly to the northern Hells Canyon area of Lake Pleasant, and we invite their presence and the sacred ceremony that is done.

We now invite the great universal goddess, Athena, into the cardinal point of the north. In through the air element and anchoring with the assistance of the north, Yei Bi Chei, and the sacred north mountain, Hesperus, the mineral of obsidian into this grid system.

We bring all that presence, inviting it into the center of the grid point at North Mountain, Eye of the Phoenix, so that Athena stands as the symbolic universal goddess. We now extend from the North Mountain, Eye of the Phoenix, connecting the sacred geometry consciousness connections directly to here, the west.

We acknowledge the Yei Bi Chei of the cardinal point—the west and the sacred mountain of the west, the San Francisco

Mountains of Flagstaff—acknowledging the mineral turquoise, the infrastructure, and the interconnection of the west to the oceans, the water element of the planet.

We invite this universal goddess energy—a form of the quantum continuum—into not only the oceans but *all* the waters, through the aggregate channels' underground passages, the irrigation systems, and even the plumbing systems connecting the quantum continuum link to the water element, allowing the quantum envelopment to seep slowly into all the infrastructures and their sacred geometry, connecting all fractured components in all beings, in all life.

We ask that it infuses the blood in the veins, arteries, and capillaries within all beings. That all beings are becoming the resonate reservoir and the quantum itself. We ask that this sacred energy be imbued into the minerals, the turquoise, and the sacred covenant of the blue corn pollen, and also into the turquoise arrowhead representing the cutting of the old infrastructures, the old third dimension, in preparation of accepting and abiding within the new quantum unstructured infrastructure.

We ask for a gentle as possible dissolution of the old so the new can be built. We ask that this ceremonial smoke then be used as the medium of this cleansing, this balancing, this healing, and this grounding into the infrastructure requested. Keep these prayers and intentions eternally sustained and ever-expanding into all beings present on this planet—all races, all divine lineages, gods, goddesses, and their associations in the past, present, and future.

We thank you, divine consciousness, and all your assistants for the opportunity to work in harmony with the universe. It is this smoke for cleansing and purifying all that the water element holds inside each and every one of us. Allow dissolution of the old and the appropriate support for the new in all creation.

When smoking the peace pipe, it is this sacred tobacco obtained from one of the four sacred mountains that was used in peace pipes before you spoke in counsel with other honored and respected beings on topics sacred in nature.

Charlie brought a rock from Ein Bokek, a town on the west coast of the Dead Sea, for placement at the power spot. This symbolically connects Israel, the sacred holy land, with the White Tanks Mountain power spot to honor the activation and the energy of this area. Both Charlie and Ron had been to Israel, where the rock was from.

Ron: I remember going to the Dead Sea just below Metsada. Arrowheads of the proper color and mineral respective to the four directions and the four sacred mountains can be used for representing the clearing and cleansing the appropriate sacred direction and any conscious or unconscious attachments to external disharmonics. Turquoise honors the Yei Bi Chei (Navajo God) of the West. Corn pollen, whether it's white, yellow, blue, or black, is used to ground in the prayer and act upon the covenant of the appropriate Yei Bi Chei of the appropriate cardinal direction.

After the ceremony, we walked back to the car. On the trail on the side of the hill, we saw four deer and stopped in our tracks to pay homage. This was auspicious, as the deer of each direction honored our intention and sacred ceremony. We felt their gratitude in our hearts. The appreciation was mutual.

When we looked up in the sky toward the rock formations we'd left, we saw the sky color and cloud formation appear as fire. This was confirmation of the message to go to Saguaro Lake, Arizona, the direction of the fire element.

Charlie departed for California to visit with friends the next morning. Then the following day, he drove from California to Arizona to visit a mentor from his younger days. While I was talking on the phone with Randy (Cherokee Indian), Charlie felt an energy blast. He took photos of the sun and said the energy came from me. I told him I was answering a question, checking my auric field, and sensing its circumference and height and form at that moment in time, and it had felt wider.

At 5:05 p.m., Charlie drove through Phoenix on I-10 and messaged me, asking if my energy was increasing. He hoped I was doing well and asked how I was. He missed my company and mentioned he'd had a wonderful visit too. He wrote that the first three adjectives that came to mind for him about me were graceful, elegant, and delicate.

On December 13, I shared a dream with Ron about standing at the crossroads of two diagonal roads. The road on the right was cloudy and dark and had buildings on both sides. The road on the left was clear blue sky and sunny, with a field of grass and no buildings. There were buildings between the two roads. My feeling at this time in the dream was that the road on the right represented the closure of the masculine energy, and the road on the left represented the opening of the feminine energy, thus giving us a peaceful and positive environment of existence in consciousness.

On Tuesday, December 15, Ron and I drove out to Saguaro Lake because of the information previously described by the fire element in the sky. Ron saw the white belly of a red-tailed hawk on the drive to the power spot as it swooped into view and made a 90-degree turn directly in front and over the car. It was quick. I was looking in another direction and had not seen the hawk. After a healthy hike up a steep climb on the side of the mountain, we reached the vista point where we could see in all four directions—the lake to the east, the Four Peaks to the north, the vast desert to the west, and the adjoining mountain to the south.

Ron spoke of the grid we'd worked on so far. The transcription of the recording is here:

We are at the Eastern power point of the grid. Formerly, we activated and did ceremony at Casa Grande, Castle Hot Springs/ Lake Pleasant, which represents the grid center pole and acts as the spine between Void and Parusha, void and consciousness. So that makes the central column pole critical.

I did not know we were even going to need to do anything more than that, but you started getting those dreams about the next spot and I was getting instructions while in my quantum meditations about the next power spots to activate.

So, in reviewing, we went to the cardinal point of the north first (after the central column). And you remember the balloon I commonly use as a metaphoric symbol modeling the archetypal, Parusha, and the void, and the void is referred to as Pakrati. So, in the balloon model, twisting it at the center demonstrates how two (Purusha & Prakriti) came from one balloon sphere. Both portions of that twisted balloon act as a "set" and hence, silver represents the void (Prakriti), but mastery of the void as in the goddess or god perspective, just as the moon represents the collective unconscious and mastery over the moon is mastery over polarized positive or polarized negative both are reflected light, so mastery over polarizations in us and others is compassionate understanding and appreciation of what polarized consciousness evolves to and promotes clear-seeing. Mastery over the moon (reflected light and its polarizations) is divinity, right?

Parusha is the non-dualistic Light of infinite compassion, so when we were working in complete surrender to spirit, allowing it to call the shots and timing, we assisted in setting that as an activation and an opening for the divine Goddess into the north of our grid's cardinal point, which is phenomenal in itself to surrender to the higher divine will. Then we observed in humility as all of the elements came together by spirit with its serendipity and in such fluidity.

We then next went to Sears-Kay Ruins and used the obsidian, which is the mineral used to honor the cardinal point of the north Yei Bi Che, Navajo Spirit, and also represents the unconscious in the human zone of consciousness. That is why we have the four directions and the center pole. The north also represents the unconscious, but in addition, it can represent the summation of all human intelligence or structured intelligence in comparison to the continuum of consciousness, which is unstructured intelligence or quantum consciousness, which is the cardinal point of the above. Human intelligence will never out-weigh or out-perform quantum consciousness as it (human intelligence) dissolves upon entering quantum consciousness.

Everything we made from our unconscious is all of the external inventions, technology, and creations we experimented with or enjoyed over lifetimes as we searched for external resolutions for our dilemmas and challenges, all of that stuff. So, knowing that, we set that understanding into the grids and that is allowing access of both poles to now move into the mind area and its unconscious creations it is still attached to. To assist in overcoming and integrating this, the mind has to be still.

So, it is necessary that quantum continuum of both the Void (Prakriti), which is unconscious quantum, and that of Purusha, which is the conscious quantum, are coming into this octa-hedronal grid consciously and hence they needed male and female of non-dualistic consciousness practiced to some degree of compassionate understanding that the shadow cannot be destroyed but integrated via non-dualistic compassion in order for the foundation to be successfully orchestrated else an over-abundance of polarized consciousness infused into the grid would have unwanted results.

As we went to the north, we invited the balanced male and female to allow the anchoring of the quantum of both to come and anchor, which stills the mind, which opened up the next step.

They had us move to the west. The element of water represents the west. They used turquoise. Coming in, this was really critical that this is the time that Athena, the date was perfect where we, who are in the astrologic planetary alignment, are the point where the gate opens to allow the divinity to come through, which is working the divine quantum consciousness. Athena, the date was perfect where we, in the astrologic, It's the point where the gate opens to allow the divinity,

So, I was intentionally making a note here between the consciousness and the intellect. The north is, let's say, the summation of all intellect. It can be divine, but it has to be merged and integrated with the unstructured quantum consciousness.

So, we opened the gate on west, which was allowing just the quantum to flow in both parts and we had the water, the clouds. We did not know what was next, but we got the direction in the dreams and they were showing me too in the quantum, instead of... I expected but did not hold that as the rule that we were going to go counterclockwise. So, I thought we were going to go south next, but they showed in the dream, go across. This was the letter Z in Barbara's dream. Z also represents spiraling.

From the quantum, intelligence, which is available as the mind is quieted, the quantum itself, communicates as quantum consciousness. Athena represents that quantum consciousness in action and she is fierce because what is she fierce about? She is fierce about not upholding any structure. Her weaponry is all about tearing down any structure. So, she stays outside the system and at times comes in to reset divine order as (and how) it is needed at that time. So, a good metaphor, the divine feminine is the dragon. The golden dragon.

Barbara: I just got something (downloaded information). Charlie, who was with us, was born in 1975 and is most likely an Indigo. They (Indigos) came in to breakdown the structures, beliefs, and programming of government, finance, politics, religion, and education. The Big 5! That's why he was there, at the west power point in the White Tanks!!

Ron laughing: It was to be revealed later! Beautiful!

Barbara: I was wondering why!? Now we know!!

Ron: Beautiful! Yes! And, he also needs, from what I can see, to be able to balance. He is so powerful as he is pure fire element! But he needs the quantum. The quantum is fluid and fluidity as it gave birth to all five elements. The first thing out of the quantum fluid was the element of fire. Fire, then, gave the motivation, gave the orchestration to create all of this, all of the structuring! I have got goosebumps! So that quantum coming into the grids needs to be invited. Do you remember I said, because we're here we can invite, we can work in association with, but we can't tell it what to do? But, when we are in harmony with it, we can invite it, it moves even quicker. It's more powerful to invite. We are here. Obviously, we have done enough of our own personal shadow work to not see any fault in any anything. The shadow is here to teach through experience and understanding to get the compassion so that it can be brought back into the quantum without judgment. It's recognized. "I need you. Thank you! Boy, were you a bastard! But I was the teacher!" But, thank you very much. It woke me up! We needed that.

The intellect (which fire is) and our direction here today is also fire. This is fire of the mind and fire of the divine. It is inviting the dragon to overcome the character's dream. So, going back to opening up the cardinal point of the north and the west in the order that we did makes so much sense because you're moderating this presiding predilection of unconscious structuring, to allow it for stillness and the arising of the new unstructured and the paradigm it is bringing into manifestation.

The Z you saw in your dream cloaks another metaphoric symbol in which Z is another example of a spiral. In the Kabala's version of the "tree of life," do you know how the energy flows within it? It makes a Z pattern. In the Kabala, you can see definite tetrahedron, then cube, then icosahedron. The tetrahedron, cube, and icosahedrons are all representative to the lower part of the tree of life or our first chakras before the heart. The tetrahedron represents grounding and survival issues, very humanistic. With the cube, you're grounding the physics of the 3-D reality and basic relationships and community, but getting ready for the icosahedron.

The icosahedron is an angular geometric form that is close to a sphere. This sphere represents the solar plexus chakra as it is the chakra where we experiment with emotions and conditional love. There is a cross-over invisible bridge, so-to-speak, from the chakra of conditional love and emotions to that of unconditional divine love and it requires complete surrender. When we surrender, we move into divine order. But below that unconditional love chakra, we have human order. It's conditional love.

So, what we are doing here now in this ceremony and activation of the cardinal direction of the east is setting the pathway and moving the merged unstructured divine and the north's unconscious structured saturnian aspect we opened and anchoring them both into the west. Now this is the gift to the world. This is the two roads that you saw in your dream.

This whole journey we are taking is so that we have the infrastructure of understanding to abide within. We are allowing that consciousness to come down to the earth. Those who can walk into and abide within that compassionate understanding are literally the Jacob's Ladder (the bridge between Heaven and Earth).

The cardinal point and gateway of the east is invoking the new paradigm. As we are giving honor to the east, we are opening the door. Each individual has to be able to enter into that themselves. That's the invitation. That's the threshold.

Tomorrow we ground all the aspects we have just described into the earth. It's the closure. As we're doing this, you're going to hear me talk about moving our full consciousness as much as we can in this moment, while we are doing the ceremony. In that way, we move our consciousness to that North Mountain and its Eye of the Phoenix vortex.

North Mountain and its Eye of the Phoenix vortex represent the absolute center of the metaphorical twist in the balloon of Purusha/Prakriti and the spine and singularity, holding the whole void and the whole of Parusha. Yes, that's the doorway, the six-sided doorway (pointing to the star opal tetrahedron pendant I was wearing). As we bring our consciousness to there and hold that fullness, we're going to repeat the invitation to each of those six cardinal points, inviting them all over here in the east.

It's time for us to consciously feel the whole and hold the whole octa-hedronal map, and with it, we add in every power spot on the planet and every fractal in every being. That is where we are going with all of this. We are acknowledging our conscious interconnectedness in all of it. The work is basically done because we understand the entire scope of what all of this is and we are allowing all of this. This is the formalization of going through the ceremony to make it finalized. Tomorrow, that will be it. That is what it is all for!

Ron said a prayer for Zeysan and the Quest ECSS [Ending Child Sex Slavery] teams. I also said a prayer for Charlie and what he was experiencing in his life, for greater peace and resolution of his challenges.

Smoking Mountain Tobacco with the peace pipe, I channeled the mathematical star language. Ron buried a yellow agate arrowhead and cornmeal into the ground with the burnt tobacco as an offering to Mother Earth and Great Spirit. A bee arrived on the peace pipe box and tobacco. Good sign!

The letter Z was another example of a spiral. The Kaballah, the tree of life. Do you know how the energy flows in it? It makes a Z pattern. In the Kaballah, you can see definite tetrahedron, then cube, then icosohedron. That was all representative to, in the lower part of the tree of life. That was survival issue, very humanistic, the chakras. Cube, you're grounding, but getting ready for icosa. The icosa was closest to a sphere. There was a cross from unconditional divine. When we surrender, we move into divine order. But below that, we have human order. It's conditional love. So, what we are doing here now, we are moving- we did the divine part, now this was the gift to the world. This was the two roads that you saw in your dream. This has to be done. We are crossing over. We are carrying them, that divine understanding and the divine spirit. It was flattening yesterday and today, carrying the energy. It's like we are going into the cube and tetrahedron tomorrow, if everything's okay, all lines up, then we go south and anchor it into the earth.

This whole journey we are taking, was so that we have the infrastructure to abide and understand. We are allowing that to come down to the earth. Those who can walk into that, are the Jacob's ladder (the bridge between Heaven and Earth). The east was the new paradigm. As we are giving honor to the east, we are opening the door. Each individual has to be able to enter into that. That's the invitation, that's the threshold. Tomorrow we ground it all into the earth. It's the closure. As we're doing this, you're going to hear me talk about we move our full consciousness, as much as we can, in this moment, while we are doing the ceremony, we move our consciousness to that North Mountain Eye of the Phoenix. That represents the absolute center of the balloons, and the spine, and the singularity, holding the whole void and the whole of Parusha.

Yes, that's the doorway, the six-sided doorway (pointing to the star opal tetrahedron pendant I was wearing). As we bring our consciousness to there, and holding that fullness, we're going to repeat the invitation to each of those areas, bringing it over to here, as we are feeling the whole, It's time for us to felt the whole and hold the whole map, every power spot on the planet, and every fractal in every being. That was where we are going with all of this. We acknowledge all of it. The work was basically done because we understand what was all of this and we are allowing all of this. This was the formalization of going through the ceremony to make if finalized. Tomorrow, that would be it. That was what it was all for!

Upon ceremony, Ron spoke of releasing the old, structured masculine and the embracing and welcoming of the unstructured feminine. As he spoke, I felt home. He mentioned the power points of Mother Earth. Just as he said that, my third eye opened, and I saw the flipping pages of a catalog of all of the Earth's power points, such as Stone Henge, Avesbury, Easter Island, Uluru (Ayers Rock in Australia), and so forth. The visual was so fast, I could not keep up with all of the images.

Ron buried a yellow agate arrowhead and cornmeal into the ground with the burnt tobacco as an offering to Mother Earth and Great Spirit. A bee arrived on the peace pipe box and tobacco. Good sign!

The next night as I laid down to allow my Higher Self to show me, they said, "As above, so below. Yesterday, as you ascended the mountain from the below of the parking lot, representing the unconsciousness, the physical reality you humans experience, you traveled upon boulders, thorns, unsteady wobbly rocks, and a steep climb representing the journey of life. You asked for Ron to help you navigate around those large boulders. Ask and you shall receive, as you are shown there are times you need assistance along the way. The larger boulders represent the advanced spiritual concepts you are attempting to embrace. This is what compassionate humans do—they help one another, for there is no separation. The journey has serendipitous moments such as finding the answer to your question about your cosmic orgasm. Ron discovered something within you he had not known, and it brought him joy.

"You were able to see your own strength and endurance in the journey up the mountain because you did not whine nor fall down. You felt our support all the way. When you reached the top of the mountain, the energy felt good. The air felt clean. You could see the environment out to the horizon, with the clarity of an eagle. The top of the mountain represents your attainment of consciousness, enlightenment, your home, your peace and comfort. This is the above, and superposition.

"Now that you and Charlie are connected energetically, his work will be magnified as the new codes have been installed within him to transmit through his intentional prayer in the electric grids, which are connected to Mother Earth's grids and the cosmic grid. You, Barbara, intentionally, with great compassion and care, gave everything you offered to Charlie so that his consciousness would be realized within him. You kept your power, allowing Charlie to experience the Divine Feminine that is soft, elegant, graceful, and delicate. At the same time, as he told you, he could feel the power within you that when called upon would be brought forward to assist as needed. This is a new reality he had never experienced before. He is in awe and still intrigued with you, as he wrote in the message he sent to you.

"Carry on. There is more to come. There is no end. There is no beginning. All there is, is love. Yes, you and Ron have had many lifetimes together in the whole human expression of duality. Isn't it a delight to have you both on a mountain top, expressing love and gratitude for each other, for all of your experiences? This is an echoing of what is in store for all of humanity stepping into the Golden Age of Peace. The evolution of the human to join cosmic brothers and sisters in the Christ Consciousness. Blessings upon Ron, upon Barbara, and upon Charlie."

We saw another hawk in the air as we traveled on the freeway to South Mountain on December 16. We hiked up to the power point that was filled with gleaming, mica-infused white quartz rocks. At the power point, Ron initiated the ceremony. In the stillness of this spot, it was peacefully quiet in the mind. I went out to the stars and saw all of the grids. At one point, my hands were on my thighs, palms up, fingers held in position as if holding Ron's two quartz balls he uses for teaching purposes. One is crystal clear, and the other is faceted. I could feel and see the balls in my hands during the meditation. After smoking the peace pipe, I channeled the mathematical star language.

There was silence, then the WhiteOne came through and spoke through my vocal cords.

The stillness is beautiful. When they show you, when you're in the experiential state, not only are you seeing but you are feeling the whole thing too, as it is grounding, they opened up the whatever, I was able to experience being Earth, being the Milky way, and also the Andromeda. From Andromeda, the connections, the superposition enacted the linkage, tick, tick, tick, tick.

Barbara: It feels so good here.

Ron: Pure nothingness. (Laughing softly.)

We smoked the peace pipe with sacred mountain smoke.

Barbara: They are showing me a pulsating point, like an antenna signal going out from here and from out there! Silence. I am out in the stars right now.

Ron (laughing): Just like that, oh my God!

Silence.

Then Ron began to channel: Acknowledging the infinite expanse of the continuum and our heart connecting to each of the galactic spirals in the expanse of the void and the quantum unicity present at their cores. We are here at the cardinal point of the southern gate and acknowledge the interlocking linkage to all things in all of creation, across the entire cosmos. We acknowledge the interconnections of all singularities to each other and the Source of Consciousness itself. This active center of all fractals with its peace, its universality, is quantum equanimity. Equally supportive and co-creative at all its junctions, connecting all beings, all structures, all creations. Acknowledging the systemic interlocking linkage and all of its fine filaments stretching across the continuum of consciousness and continuum of the void where all things are created.

From this consciousness, we walk with it through all its connections, acknowledging this presence, this equanimity of physicality and spirit, into the center of the North Mountain Eye of the Phoenix. As we acknowledge the Eye of the Phoenix presence as an access way from the quantum continuum, permeating in all directions, we anchor this southern cardinal point branch of consciousness with that of the center pole.

Next, we add the Casa Grande symbolic metaphor stretching across the entire void and rising as a single pole straight through the Eye of the Phoenix into the heart of Purusha as the continuum of consciousness. We link now the center pole with the Castle Hot Springs/Lake Pleasant cardinal point of the above and the Sears-Kay-North, White Tank Mountains-West, Saguaro Lake Cardinal point-East, spiraling down to here, South Mountain.

The whole structure has been walked, prayed, lived, blessed, and integrated by the two intertwining male and female aspects of our two consciousness, acting as the One, in non-duality.

Receptive of compassionate understanding and appreciative of the clear seeing of joy, acknowledgment, and validation of love. You each have walked and ground the whole of existence into this metaphoric archetypal grid system, shared, enacted, instigated, inspired, into the fractals and all of the power spots all across the planet, all across the solar system now, all across the universe and within all beings. All the gifts, awakenings, understandings, returned to the fractal of Source within all beings, emphasizing the inner map and guide's capacity for healing the wholeness. Heal the self to let go of the self-stewarding and dissolving into the One-Source. That is the infrastructure that supports the conscious transition from being the dense character, animal, reptile, insect of primordial consciousness in all of its phases to now holding the Divine ready to dissolve separation itself.

Now, the door is open. And with the opening of the door, releasing all the stored charges, allow them to return to the black quantum of unconsciousness, return to Black Lilith, giving thanks, for without her separation is impossible, impossible to experience limitations. The wound creates compassion and awakening, but now after awakening we return what is borrowed as unconsciousness and limitation must be returned.

In this new infrastructure and grid activation, it promotes the purging and the healing, directing all those old wounds to return to the mother of all wounds, Black Lilith. The mother of separation reality supports our return to our original wholeness.

Her aspects of time, experience, limitations, contraction, repulsion with all the stratifications of irrationality and alienation, that illusion she provided is now over. And so, we impart an infinite pathway to consciousness, to compassion and integration, within the fractals in all beings and in all separation states of consciousness by the activation of this octa-hedronal grid and its connection to all nodal points of all the consciousness grids on this planet.

In all lineages, in all timelines, all the sacred directions, the use of this space, this time, these areas, are for the purpose of giving back and blessing all life with this map, and so we honor all the sacrifices that have gone before to make this moment full of blessed empowerment. With these ceremonies and activations may they now serve as connection to all beings to return all structure, all consciousness, all particles, all beings, back to the peace, fulfillment and stillness of quantum equanimity and superposition.

So we ask all the beings and legions of light from the heart center of Divine Creation, the heart center of Divine Purusha, for your presence, participation, and assistance in holding, grounding, purifying, balancing, and healing all the inter-connected lines of consciousness that ties us within you, you within us, in the sacred six directions of the North, South, East, West, Above and Below.

We ask you attend to these within the physical body, mental body, emotional body, conscious body, astral body on all densities and dimensional levels for all beings on this planet. The emanation of this intention, energy and prayers from this moment forward for all beings, we ask your presence in this smoke, a final cleansing, purifying, healing, balancing, and grounding take place in all beings, all races, all guardians, all gods, guides, and we thank you.

I began speaking the mathematical star language, then the WhiteOne came forward and said, "Goodness Gracious, Dear Ones! We knew you were waiting for us. We love dear Ron! He is such a delight for us to view, hear, feel. God Bless you both indeed! For this journey of time and effort, energy, heart, compassion, intention, consciousness, all of it, dear friends, we are very grateful. What you have done for all of humanity and for all of the cosmos and especially for Mother Earth. She is very, very pleased with your assistance because as you are of the Oneness that she is, it is such a comprehensive and additive exponential component, if you will, of the ceremony, of the change, of the codes, of the activation, of the de-activation, and for the evolution that is occurring here and there and everywhere.

For as you evolve, so do others. God Bless you indeed. You've done great work. You hold the energy. You hold the codes. Dear Ron and dear Barbara, for this work and for the individual work you do with people and groups and others in the room, and so with this qualification of two with great compassion and unconditional love and a high understanding, an advanced understanding of this purpose of ceremony, of concepts, we are very grateful that you have agreed to participate in the flux and the change in the Ascension. God Bless you indeed. That is all.

Ron: Thank you, WhiteOne.

I felt sublime peace and love as I climbed down the mountain with Ron. He later shared with me that as we were walking down, he noticed that it was so quiet. I wasn't talking, and he had thought to himself, *This is not like Barbara.* He had turned around and exclaimed at that moment, "Oh my God, the energy is so peaceful!"

I'd said, "I can't even speak!"

CHAPTER 20

Quantum Navigation Journeys

THIS GRID WORK FOR HUMANITY had to be completed before the Winter Equinox on December 21, 2020. We completed this mission over a three-week period. Ron told me that we were now stewards of the grid and must monitor it and make energetic adjustments as needed. I was given a visual by the quantum navigator to determine the condition and structure of the grid. I am able to do this monitoring remotely. If we receive information to physically go to any point on the grid, we will inform one another. The quantum navigator gave me more information in subsequent meditations.

During a Quantum Navigator Meditation group with Ron Holt using Zoom, this was what I experienced. I saw a golden light bathing my body, clearing my chakras, and healing my body. Standing in front of a huge turbine engine/generator of a power plant in a very large building, I noticed the blades of the engine were made of faceted aquamarine stones. They were a medium blue and very large. Aquamarine is the birthstone of March. There was a large hole in the middle of the engine apparatus, and I was instructed to enter the engine through that hole. I was sitting in a lotus position, floating into the engine. Once inside the engine, I said to myself, "Wait, this isn't an engine. It's a portal!" (I was actually delighted to be given this form of visual and vehicle for me to travel through.)

I began traveling through a wormhole into outer space and looked back, seeing Earth moving very fast in the opposite position. Then

I saw the Milky Way galaxy fading away into the distance. I turned around and saw myself approaching the Great Central Sun.

I went into the sun, then was located in the middle of the star, standing in a huge "monitoring room." There were consoles along the walls, and beings of various kinds were working. I was shown a display in the middle of the room that had a shallow glass dome. I estimated the diameter to be about five to six feet across. Looking into the dome, I saw the Eye of Phoenix power grid in Arizona. It brought up an immense amount of emotion, so much that I physically cried. (Feeling emotion in the theta state means a person is deep). I was feeling unconditional love, gratitude, and the enormity of the energy work we did for Earth, humanity, and the universe.

The beings (Quantum Navigator/Higher Self collective) showed me the Earth grid below, the electric grid that Charlie works on, and the cosmic grid. In the display, there were light beams traveling from each point and connecting to other points. When there was a disturbance in the grids, it would show up as either a change in the color of the light beam or a variance in the intensity of the light. When that occurred, the beings were able to send a message to the beings connected to the grids, to check in, connect, and raise the vibration or modulate the frequency for optimum function. From this monitoring room, humans were assisted on Earth. I was told I would be given more information, but this was the end of what the QN wanted to show me for now.

I washed my face and returned to meditation on the sofa, where a blue light bathed my body from above. I saw a wormhole and traveled through it. Going through other wormholes connecting the universes, the color of the wormhole entrances/exits was vibrant: reds, yellows, oranges, blues, and greens. Then, I was plopped on a sofa on a lunar surface. I'd done this before. The QN said, "Now, instead of viewing Mother Earth, we want you to view this, the entire cosmos, as the observer."

At home, during a meditation at 6:00 a.m., my Higher Self again showed me the Great Central Sun "monitoring room." I saw the components of the room and the beings turned into descending ones and zeroes, like in the *Matrix* movie. I was inside a computer program. The components turned back into the images as before.

I asked, "What was the point of everything? Why?"

They removed everything from my sight and told me, "Now there is nothing. We now ask you, Barbara, why not?"

I replied, "This is profound. Yes, why not all of this?"

They said to me, "Where there is nothing, there is not. The word and concept of not is in the word nothing. No-thing. Not-thing. Here is in there. Here is in where. Wherever. Where is everything. Ever comprises everything, everywhere, everlasting. No beginning. No end. It just is. Now, you have a profound appreciation for All That Is—an immense appreciation for all of your experiences, the entire world experiences, and the entire universe experiences. Contemplate, dear one."

In a subsequent meditation, Ron and I were in a high-rise office building many floors up, sitting around a table with other people, and Ron was teaching. Ron kept looking at me, and I was nodding my head in agreement with what he said to us. I walked over to the glassless window in the wall of 1.5-inch-thick concrete up to my waist. When I leaned out the window, I looked down and became physically shocked that the ground was so far away. We were really high up, hundreds of floors above the ground. There was a beautiful turquoise crystal-clear river, and the surrounding environment was a light beige color. It was very clean-looking. No garbage, no debris, nothing dark.

The office building represented our inner work. The height of the building represented the level of consciousness. The absence of a window represented no obstacles whatsoever because the window portrayed the quality and quantity of personal perception. The clean environment represented the condition of the landscape of our consciousness.

During a quantum navigation gathering with Ron via a video platform, I went into meditation. First, I was floating as consciousness in fluidity. I rocked back and forth, very gently and very lovingly. I was shown a white owl and taken back to the west power point in the grid at the White Tanks Regional Park. There, I was standing at the ceremony spot, holding hands with Charlie. I effortlessly placed my left hand into the ground where the stones were buried. Elevated on a nearby rock, Ron sat in meditation with his eyes closed. I saw a large, six-foot-long white feather before me. The tip was pointing toward the ground. The feather morphed into a fan of white feathers. It became apparent to me that this was a ceremonial feather fan on the back of some person, as part of their regalia. The person moving the fan turned around. The head was an eagle, and I recognized Chief White Eagle. He began to dance. As soon as his legs moved up and down, I was filled with an immense amount of love. At the same time, I was feeling all of the anguish and pain of humanity, feeling all of the mental and emotional wounds. Tears were streaming down my face as I sat on the sofa in my apartment.

After a minute of tears, I saw a series of metallic triangles suspended in the air above me with the cosmos as a backdrop. The material the triangles were made of was not of this Earth. I flew through the triangles, out into the cosmos, and traveled among the stars and planets. The scene transitioned to me deep in a tower of turquoise blue water. I swam upward, toward the light at the top of the tower. When I reached the surface of the water, I crawled out and onto a platform with a railing. My fellow meditators were with me, including Ron. Looking out to the horizon, I could see the Florida coastline and the Atlantic Ocean. I suddenly realized we were at Cape Canaveral, on top of a Saturn V rocket launch pad. The black nose cone of the rocket opened up like a clamshell. We saw five seats and climbed into the seats, then the cone closed. I realized at this moment that we were going to be launched into space. The rocket took off, and we began our space travel. My alarm rang for the conclusion of the meditation time.

Ron commented, "The west point of the grid represents, in Navajo tradition, the Pacific Ocean and bringing in water for the fluidity. Pallas Athena is the eternal virgin. She was born from the head of Zeus, fully formed. She is not from the earth. She retains her originality, her quantum goddessness. She's never been diminished. She was born whole. She remains outside of the system. She stays organically pure. When she comes into the system, *wow*! She is fierce because she reorganizes things back to their original template and divine orientation.

"As we were opening that gate, I got that was your hand in the ground with all of the elements we used to help honor the gods of that direction in alignment with the goddess coming in. That was the invitation for her to come in, as the fluidity to absolve, resolve, and dissolve—that capacity to come into the grid that is changing from the old patriarchal to now. I didn't care what your story is. Let's just get back to divine fluidity. This is what that ceremony was all about.

"All the ceremonies we did were in honor of Grandfather White Eagle. He was acknowledging it in another way. The work we did, did its job. The white feathers are a representation of Saraswati. Her signet was also the owl. She is the deity with the many arms that rides on the back of an owl. She orchestrates all the structure by her song. When we are ready to go back into nothingness, she sings and dissolves us all back. Grandfather White Eagle is the gatekeeper of that energy. His big thing is bringing all of the strands of all of the races into one tapestry. The only way those strands come together in the tapestry is when one honors that process. The Tower card in the Tarot shatters all of the structure so that you remain fully vulnerable and malleable. Only when all of the structure is taken away can you return to your true essence—no ego-based posturing, tension, or structure. In that fluidity, those drops of consciousness can come together. All past identifiers that the character holds, such as shame, blame, fear, and guilt, are ways we view ourselves. We misidentify our original fabric by the entanglements we've held for so long, so we've got to let them go.

"You can hold the grid. We were asked to. In holding the grid, you make no stories of everybody else, letting go of all of their stuff to give back to Black Lilith. Being in that state, not holding onto any story, being in that quantum fluidity, you moved through all these gates to wherever consciousness wants to take you. Consciousness wants you to participate in this. This is the absolution of any structure. You are being invited to explore consciousness for your next book. This will get you through all the gateways represented by those series of triangles. You will keep returning to yourself as you go through the gateways in your explorations. You will not get lost. The quantum fluidity will take anything thrown at it and dissolve it into love. The love is deep and vast. You experienced it."

I pulled the Integrity card of the Galactic Heritage card deck, and Ron said this was all me, what I had experienced. There is nothing higher than integrity. Integrity is unconditional love. You can't get to integration without the root word "integrity."

I also pulled a card from the Osho card deck and was given the Friendliness card. Depicted on the card were two trees representing the yin and yang, our paradoxical dualism. Not polarized duality. Rather, we are an infinite collection of equal opposites. The horseshoe magnets are no longer in repulsion but now in attraction. This is integration. There is no judgment lying in between the dualities, only conscious awareness. There is compassionate understanding and clear seeing. There is no conscious opposition and nothing to manifest, so they disappear. They want to take you rapidly through those thresholds you saw as the triangles.

Magnificent, fluid, and diamond clear! I could now see this beautiful orchestration to the ending of the grid work, combined with an invitation to expand my consciousness through further journeys into the quantum field. I go eagerly into the next phase of my life. I hope my readers are able to take the concepts and apply them to their own lives, experiences, and the unconditional love the universe holds for them.

I have gone through a massive amount of growth and evolution of my spirituality and consciousness since 2012. The journey continues out into the cosmos and the quantum field, the subject of my next QHHT® session stories book. I invite you to join me as we explore interstellar, transdimensional travel through Quantum Healing Hypnosis Technique℠ sessions in my next book, *Star Travels: Exploration of Interdimensional Interstellar Transport.*

BOOKS BY BARBARA BECKER

Enclosure: A Spiritual Autobiography

Expansion: The Journey Continues

Time Travels: Exploration of Lives Remembered

A SNEAK PEEK OF

Enclosure:
A Spiritual Autobiography

CHAPTER 1

My Out-of-Body Experience

U NTIL AGE THIRTY-ONE, I HAD been blessed with a relatively healthy body. I had the usual childhood illnesses—occasional colds and flu bugs. I didn't have weight issues or a desire to abuse alcohol or smoke tobacco. But one evening I sustained a serious injury that put me in the place of one of my critically injured patients.

In June of 1986, I met the man who would become my second husband, Hoyt L. Kesterson, II. He had wanted to date me for two years. When I ended a relationship with another man, Hoyt invited me over to his home for a swim in his pool and to watch a laser disc movie of my choice from his six-hundred-disc collection.

I drove over to his house and changed into my bathing suit in the guest bathroom. When I walked outside to the patio, I saw a crystal wine bucket and two wineglasses on the pool deck. My first thought was, *Wow, this is romantic, and I don't have any romantic feelings for this man.*

He asked me what wine I'd like, and I picked white zinfandel. We sat in the pool, on the steps, talking about life and sipping wine. After swimming, he gave me his terrycloth bathrobe to wear over my suit as we watched two movies in the living room. I noticed there were several cats walking around the house, checking me out. After the second movie, I got dressed and drove to my parents' house, where I had been pet-sitting their two cats while they were in California, picking up my sister from Stanford University for the summer break.

Hoyt called the next day and asked me out for dinner and a movie with a couple of his friends. I had never gone out to dinner with three men at the same time. But all three were friends of my family, and they worked in the computer business, so I accepted the invitation.

On the morning of the date, while taking my shower, I heard two loud bang sounds in my head. I didn't think nothing much of them. I felt delighted to share a dinner with three very brilliant men with golden hearts. We watched *Legal Eagles* and later ate at the Oscar Taylor restaurant at the Biltmore Fashion Park Mall in central Phoenix.

I offered to drive us in my new, seventeen-day-old gray Honda Accord. At the time, Hoyt drove a Yamaha 1100-cc motorcycle. On the way home, he asked me to drive on Missouri Avenue so he could stop at his bank's ATM to withdraw some money.

When we entered the intersection at Seventh Street, the last thing Hoyt said to me was, "You're a good driver. Oh, oh, she's coming through!"

A woman who had been drinking and was driving a large Oldsmobile sped through a red light and hit my car, just in front of the steering wheel. The strange sounds I had heard in the shower that morning were the sounds of that large Oldsmobile hitting my Honda Accord LX and causing it to fly through a chain-link fence. I hadn't realized that morning that I'd received a clairaudient premonition of the accident.

The driver of the Olds was angry at her husband, who had been driving. He had stopped the vehicle and gotten out. She had taken off, speeding through red lights, with her twelve-year-old daughter in the passenger seat. Just as she was traveling through the intersection, I looked to my left and saw her car in slow motion—coming toward me. Upon impact, my car went airborne, broke through the chain-link fence, and landed on a four-foot dirt mound at an excavation site on the corner.

When we landed, the thoughts running through my mind were, *I'm not finished. It's not my time to die. I'm here for my sister Valerie.* Hoyt, who wasn't wearing his seat belt, landed on the floor in front of his seat. He had upper and mid-back pain, and his right leg was hurting from hitting the dashboard. But he fared better than I did. Both of my lungs were collapsed because my collarbones were snapped in half. Hoyt's two-hundred-plus-pound body had flown across the car and into my one-hundred-eighteen-pound frame. Objects move in the opposite direction of force, and I just happened to be in his path. Five of my ribs were fractured on the right side. I also had glass in my eyes from the shattered windshield.

Luckily, this accident occurred in front of a fire station, so the emergency response time was almost immediate. People stopped their cars and rushed over to us. The paramedics pulled up in their fire trucks and saw how smashed up the cars were. The windshield was shattered, mostly on the driver's side, so it looked like I had hit it with my head.

"She's got a head injury!" the paramedic shouted when he saw red liquid dripping down my forehead, mistaking it for blood.

I reached up and pulled a strawberry off my head. "It's a strawberry. I didn't hit my head." My dessert, which had been in a Styrofoam container on the dashboard, was now all over the car. The photos taken by the accident investigator later showed what looked like lung tissue and blood in the interior of the car. But it was really cake, whipped cream, and smashed strawberries.

I could talk only in short sentences because it was hard for me to breathe—like breathing in the second dimension, without expansion. I knew I was in shock because I kept repeating, "He's allergic to penicillin, and I've got contact lenses in my eyes." I was afraid I was going to go unconscious and not be in control of the situation. I couldn't stop being a critical care nurse.

The paramedics told me to climb out of the vehicle myself and crawl onto the backboard. I was surprised they couldn't lift or help to lift my body out of the vehicle. I moved in excruciating pain from the broken bones touching the nerves as I exited the vehicle by myself.

As she strapped me down on the backboard on the ground, a female paramedic told me she would have to put a MAST suit on me because my blood pressure was low and for precautionary measures for shock. I remembered that the only people I saw in the ER with a MAST suit on were dead, and they had messed their pants. This was a message for me that I was in deep doo-doo.

But then the paramedic added, "We're not going to inflate the MAST suit; we just want to be prepared." This made me feel a little bit better.

It took the paramedics several attempts to start an IV in my arms. My large veins must have been closed down with adrenalin surging through my bloodstream to keep me conscious. We were loaded into an ambulance and taken to John C. Lincoln Hospital, where I had learned how to become an ER nurse eight years before.

It was estimated the other driver was traveling about sixty miles per hour at the moment of impact, due to the two-foot intrusion into my vehicle. She hadn't applied her brakes, which caused her to receive facial injuries, smashing her front teeth out on the steering wheel. Her daughter in the passenger seat sustained injuries to both knees from the dashboard impact. They were taken by ambulance to the same hospital.

The trauma team was waiting for our arrival. As soon as I was placed on the hospital gurney, the nurses cut away my favorite V-neck sweater top and my white cotton pants and undergarments. I was covered with a sheet and a warm, light blanket. The nurses placed a catheter into my bladder to monitor my urine output. My blood was drawn for lab tests and to check my alcohol level, which turned out to be zero, even though I had one Amaretto and cola with my meal.

When the trauma nurse attempted twice to put the stomach tube into my nose and down through my throat to suck out my dinner, my body rose up off the gurney and my nails sunk into the skin of her arm. My gag reflex was trying to keep the tube from going down. Finally, she was able to insert the tube on the third try.

Every time I moved my body, I felt unbearable pain. Trauma protocol dictates that doctors withhold pain drugs until they determine the extent of the injuries so narcotic effects don't cover up a life-threatening injury. Computerized tomography scans were taken of my abdomen to rule out internal injury. The pain from my broken ribs and collarbones shot down to my abdomen. After the doctor read the negative CT scan results, the trauma nurse took the stomach tube out.

The radiology tech burst through the ER doors, yelling, "She's got bilateral pneumos!"

The trauma nurse attending to me yelled back, "She's a nurse. She knows what you're talking about!"

I imagined she thought I would freak out. But I already knew I was in serious shape when the paramedic told her at my bedside that my respiratory rate was forty-four per minute. The norm is twelve to eighteen. That's when I understood there was a serious problem with my lungs. Being a critical care nurse, and because of my personality, I kept my cool and tried not to let on how nervous I was. I was scared that I might have a torn aorta that wasn't being picked up in the tests.

A trauma surgeon came to my bedside, introduced himself, and said I needed a chest tube to reinflate my right lung. I was diagnosed with a 50 percent hemorrhage and deflation of that lung. The left lung was collapsed about 10 percent and didn't require a chest tube. The nurses set up a sterile field for the procedure after the trauma surgeon performed his exam. He injected lidocaine into my right side to numb the skin. Then he made a small incision with a scalpel, where he injected the numbing medicine, blotted the blood away, then attempted to insert the tube. The chest tube is a semihard plastic tube with a metal spear inside, like a shish kebab skewer, with the diameter just larger than the size of a pencil. The skewer, better known as a trocar, has a sharp point to facilitate piercing through the muscle fascia.

The lidocaine did nothing for the pain. I was in so much pain, my muscles were tightened. The chest tube would not go in, and consequently my whole body was pushed across the gurney. This ignited my nerve fibers so much I began to scream obscenities at the top of my lungs. "Shit! Goddamn!" I couldn't hold the words back. At the same time I was yelling these cuss words, I was thinking Hoyt could hear me and he wouldn't want to go out with me again. But there was nothing I could do to stop screaming those words.

The trauma surgeon stepped back. The nurses readjusted me back on the gurney. He tried inserting the tube again, shoving me across the gurney. "Shit! Goddamn!" I grabbed my chest with my left hand, contaminating the sterile field. I screamed at the nurses, "Tie me down! I'm touching the sterile field!"

I could see in my third eye a list of the ten complications of a trocar chest tube insertion. I knew too much. I was very afraid the spear would slip and my heart, lung, liver, or spleen would be pierced like a piece of meat on a fork, and I would die. I was totally freaking out in the most excruciating pain and in the most intense fear I'd ever felt in my life. Gauging my level of pain, I promised God I would never complain about my menstrual cramps again.

On the third try, the tube was successfully inserted. The surgeon placed it deep inside to suck up the blood and the escaped air to allow my lung to reinflate over time. When this procedure was done, I was given a shot of Demerol for the pain.

Friends took Hoyt home, and I was admitted to the hospital intensive care unit. I received pain shots every four hours around the clock. Breathing treatments with a small nebulizer were given to me to prevent pneumonia and help my lungs reinflate. During one of these breathing treatments, I read my EKG monitor backward in my mirror on the overbed table and discovered my P-wave was missing. My heart was in a junctional rhythm. Although this wasn't life threatening, I felt the trauma surgeon should be aware of it. When the respiratory tech told the trauma doctor about the cardiac rhythm anomaly, the bronchodilator drug was discontinued.

On the third day, I was transferred to the telemetry unit for close observation. This is when I began reliving the accident. During these attacks, my heart rate jumped and my hands were wet with sweat. The nurses gave me pain medication for these events.

My parents came home during my fourth day in the hospital and got the message from my brothers that I was in intensive care. My mother broke down in tears. When they visited, my sister Maureen brought flowers and could see I was alive and well, considering the circumstances. On the fifth day, I was transferred to the regular floor. My bladder catheter was removed, but I still had the chest tube.

The day after the accident, Hoyt had to leave on a business trip in New England to defend the United States' position on a computer security protocol. This was a project he and his committee had been working on for two years. If he hadn't shown up, the United States would have lost the vote. He traveled in pain and was still able to perform his job.

Before he left, Hoyt sent me the largest bouquet of flowers I've ever seen a patient receive in a hospital. The nurses showed me them from the doorway, because flowers weren't allowed at the bedside in critical care units due to possible bugs transmitting diseases, and the limited shelf space for supplies and equipment.

The trauma surgeon removed my chest tube in the afternoon of the fifth day. My lungs had reinflated to 90 percent. If someone asks me if I know what a chest tube feels like with broken ribs, I can tell them. When you lie still and the tube isn't moved by anyone, at the point where the tube is inserted, and the surrounding two inches of skin, it feels like a blowtorch is under the surface. This sensation is constant. When the tube is moved, it feels like a knife is inside your heart, twisting back and forth. From this experience, I gained more empathy for people with chest trauma.

After a week in the hospital, I continued my healing in an electrical hospital bed at my parents' home for a month. I went back to work six weeks after the accident. I worked for two days with a shoulder muscle spasm. But when my right arm went numb and cold, I called the orthopedic surgeon assigned to my case and asked for four weeks of physical therapy. I made a complete recovery in ten weeks.

While recuperating, I noticed a part of my consciousness would separate from my mind and ask questions: *Why? Why are we here? Why are we having a conversation? Why is there a sofa? A chair? Why?* Everything appeared foreign to me. These episodes would occur when I was in conversation with people and when I was by myself, and they lasted for about one or two minutes. In the beginning this happened about five times a day. It scared me because I had no control over it. I wondered if I was going insane. I didn't realize I was having out-of-body experiences.

After several days, I decided to go with it. I would say in my mind,

Oh well, here we go again. I no longer feared it. I figured it was what my mind had to do to cope with the trauma of a near-fatal accident. I didn't tell anyone about what I was going through.

These episodes gradually diminished in frequency and finally stopped after eight months. During this posttraumatic period, I didn't care if my bills were paid. I didn't care if I was on time for appointments. I was shocked at myself for feeling and behaving like this. At the time, my attitude was, *Hey, I'm not even supposed to be here.* And this perspective shocked me too. I just didn't care what people thought about me. Eventually, I became responsible again. I just figured this was how my mind dealt with the trauma.

Years later, two psychologists told me they had never heard of these types of experiences. When reading Joel Goldsmith's *The Art of Spiritual Healing*, I received a downloaded message that the portion of my consciousness that separated from me was my Higher Consciousness. Although it felt like a separation, it really wasn't. I was feeling the presence of my Higher Self. For brief moments, I pierced the veil of forgetfulness. My consciousness and awareness were being adjusted. For what, I didn't know at the time.

I was beginning to see my life changing directions. I started a relationship with Hoyt that turned into love. Within five months, he asked me to marry him. Actually, he first wanted me to move in with him. I said I would, if he agreed to marry me. After a fifteen-month courtship, we were married at the edge of the Grand Canyon in a small ceremony at Shoshone Point on September 5, 1987. It was filmed by a television company from London, Thames Television. As part of a travel show called *Wish You Were Here...?*, presented by the British actress Anneka Rice, our wedding was viewed by over thirteen million people in the United Kingdom.

Hoyt and I settled down to married life with travel and adventure. I worked at a small, local hospital part time in the emergency room, and he continued his computer standards work at Honeywell. During our eighteen-year marriage, we traveled to thirteen countries, and I was introduced to many cultures and customs. I am grateful for Hoyt giving me the world and the opportunity to begin my exploration of my spirituality.

Ten years later, at age forty-two, I began my conscious spiritual journey when I met my guardian angel.

ACKNOWLEDGMENTS

My infinite love and gratitude continues for Grandmaster Zeysan, Ron Holt, Charlie Wolfe, Shaman Lance Heard, Ann Albers, Hoyt L. Kesterson II, Peter Nufer, Candace Craw-Goldman, Grandma Chandra, Devara Thunderbeat, Maureen J. St. Germain, Lisa Montgomery, Rose Mis, Mark Johnson, Randy Bayless, Rev. Liz Johnson, Dr. Harmony, Shawn Warwick, DC, Rose Butler, Anita Robeson, Crystal Andasola, Cansu Bulgu, Nicolette Napier Froelicher, Julie Rae, Dolores Cannon, Summer Bacon, Dr. Peebles, Liz Kuester, my human family, and my star family.

ABOUT THE AUTHOR

Barbara Becker was born in Upstate New York and graduated from Glendale Community College in Glendale, Arizona with an associate's degree in Nursing. Specializing in surgical intensive care nursing, she broadened her skills in cardiac care and general critical care and emergency medicine. She was employed as the Nursing Education Director for a local Phoenix, Arizona hospital before pursuing a career in legal nurse consulting. She attained her bachelor's degree in Business Administration from the University of Phoenix. After twenty-two years in the legal field and forty years in the medical field and offering her energy healing services to individuals and groups, Barbara became a Quantum Healing Hypnosis Technique (QHHT®) practitioner.

She soon discovered a love for writing books and stories when she was urged by her Higher Self to write her autobiography. Self-taught, Barbara wrote and self-published a QHHT® session stories book to help people understand their life purpose and their ability to heal themselves.

Barbara's hobbies include hiking, camping, cooking, gardening, reading books, sewing, needlepoint, and traveling.

CPSIA information can be obtained
at www.ICGtesting.com
Printed in the USA
BVHW070120030921
615904BV00013B/1455